A-Z
of
HOSPICE
and
PALLIATIVE
MEDICINE

Peter Kaye

MA MB BChir MRCP MRCGP DRCOG

CONSULTANT IN PALLIATIVE MEDICINE, NORTHAMPTON

This book is available from:

EPL Publications
41 Park Avenue North
Northampton NN3 2HT
ENGLAND

Price £21.50, plus £1.90 post and package. Books sent by return on receipt of cheque, payable to EPL publications. (10% discount for orders of six books or more).

ISBN 0–9519895–0–2

First published 1992
Revised reprint 1994
Reprinted 1996

British Library Cataloguing-in-Publication Data
A Catalogue record for this book is available from the British Library

Typeset by Land & Unwin (Data Sciences) Ltd.,
Bugbrooke, Northamptonshire.

DEDICATED TO MY PARENTS

JOHN AND GLADYS

CONTENTS

Foreword

Anyone who has taken time to listen to a patient with far advanced disease must have heard the plea, "I knew I needed attention." So many have realized that those involved with their treatment at an earlier stage have finally implied "There is nothing more I can do." At no time has personal concern been useless but how much less true is it now after the decades of experience, research and teaching so carefully summarized in this book. Once cure has become impossible there is still a great deal that can be done. A detailed description of this potential for help, which should be always available, is presented here.

Hospice and palliative care includes much more than an understanding of symptoms and their skilled relief. It is concerned with the whole person, part of the family network who share in all the emotional, social and spiritual distress that accompany physical problems and the inexorable losses that make up the experience of mortal illness and this other dimension is also addressed here in an approachable way.

What has been learned with a solid and growing basis of research in this whole field has been largely focused on advanced malignant disease. However, the symptom control and the attitudes presented here have a much wider relevance and are increasingly interpreted in other settings and for people with different diagnoses. This book should appear in every ward reference shelf and in every Health Centre library as well as with every hospice or palliative care team.

There is another, even more important implication. As we face all the challenges of hospice and palliative care we are not the final focus of either attention or achievement. The real challenge is faced by the patient and the family group who may then be enabled to take the opportunity to use creatively what is often seen as the most important part of their life together. Once we have begun to relieve and understand the complex distress which can be overwhelming, it is they who have the chance to find growth and deeper understanding through loss. No one with Peter Kaye's experience is easily idealistic about these challenges, but confidence not only in the skills described but also in the person with the problems they present, is the essential message of this important source book.

Dame Cicely Saunders, OM., DBE.

October 1992

This book is intended for:

   — Hospice staff
   — General Practitioners
   — Macmillan nurses
   — District nurses
   — Hospital doctors
   — Specialist nurses
   — Therapists

and all professional carers of patients who are facing advanced illness, especially advanced cancer, motor neurone disease and AIDS, whether in a hospital ward, at home or in a hospice. Hopefully it will also be useful to the many people now involved in teaching palliative medicine.

This is a problem-orientated book and the information has been arranged alphabetically, to make it as accessible as possible. If you have any criticisms or suggestions about how to improve the book, I would be <u>very</u> pleased to receive them.

I have attempted to provide a summary of good practice. However, all medical care, and particularly hospice care, flows through relationships, and depends most importantly on the quality of human interactions. This aspect of care is harder to summarize. I have attempted to describe what is needed in some of the sections in the book, such as those on Counselling, Family support, Spiritual pain and Talking with the patient.

The sections on individual cancers provide a summary of useful background information, but are not intended to be a definitive statement about the management of individual cancers.

Selected references and suggestions for further reading have been included at the end of some of the sections, as a means to further study, and have usually been included because they contain a list of references for further study.

The index includes drugs under both generic (chemical) and proprietary (trade) names. <u>Abbreviations</u> are also explained in the index.

Appendices on <u>Useful Equipment</u> and <u>Useful Drugs</u> have been included at the back of the book, but are not indexed.

3 words need to be clearly defined because there is often confusion about them: Palliative, Hospice and Terminal.

Palliative care is no longer intended to be curative, but aims to control symptoms and prolong life, and may include such measures as surgery, radiotherapy or chemotherapy. 50% of cancer patients are not curable at diagnosis.

Hospice care denotes a style of care, rather than a place. Hospice care focuses on relieving symptoms and improving the quality of remaining life (including mental, social and spiritual life) and aims to meet the complex and changing needs of the patient and the family. This requires a multi-disciplinary team approach.

Terminal care is needed during the last few days of life. The family's needs are especially important at this stage. The terminal phase is characterized by day-to-day deterioration in the patient's condition.

I would like to thank the following for their helpful comments: Penny Atkinson, Sue Beresford, Nigel Bird, Pat Cooke, John Kearsey, Tess Kennedy, Len Lunn, Craig MacMillan, Barbara Malcomson, William Miers, Mike Severn, Liz Starmer, Ann Taylor-Chiltern and Jo Warcaba. I would also like to thank Ann Skinner and her staff at the Cripps Medical Centre library for their help with finding references. Finally, I want to express my sincere thanks to Gill Hervey-Murray for her encouragement and support.

Revised Reprint 1994. Significant changes have been made to the section on Dyspnoea. Minor additions or amendments have also been made to the sections on AIDS, Ascites, Bleeding, Bone Pain, Colon cancer, Dysphagia, Hiccup, Hormone therapy, Intestinal obstruction, Laxatives, Morphine, Motor Neurone Disease, Nerve pain, NSAIDS, Prostate cancer, Steroids and Subcutaneous infusions. Some important new references have been added. I am grateful to Michael Mower and others for pointing out typing and spelling errors. Despite my best efforts, errors may still have occurred – as with all medical books, check all figures and doses.

Peter Kaye
Cynthia Spencer House
Northampton
England

January 1994

Principles of Symptom Control

The 12 common symptoms are:

- Weakness   82%
- Dry mouth   68%
- Anorexia   58%
- Depression   52%
- Insomnia   46%
- Pain   46%
- Swollen legs   46%
- Nausea   42%
- Constipation   36%
- Vomiting   32%
- Confusion   30%
- Dyspnoea   30%

This list comes from a survey by an Australian medical student of hospice and hospital patients with advanced cancer, who were asked to select cards with symptoms written on them. The average number of symptoms was 7. Note that pain is no longer the main problem. (Dunlop GM, Palliative Medicine 1989, 4: 37-43).

Symptom control is straightforward. It is possible to reduce physical distress in all patients and to keep most patients free of symptoms. The method of controlling symptoms is the same as that of routine diagnosis: history, examination and occasionally special tests (e.g. serum calcium in nausea).

Formal enquiry is necessary, because most patients have several symptoms (*see Assessment* for symptom list). Ask "Why?". It is essential to consider why the symptom is occuring (why is the patient vomiting, breathless etc.) so that reversible causes can be be treated and medication can be specific

The examination for physical signs (oral thrush, pleural effusion, bony tenderness, hepatomegaly, impacted faeces) is also an opportunity to raise a patient's morale. Touch can be powerfully therapeutic and it can also be very encouraging to the patient if the doctor says something positive e.g. "Your lungs sound healthy".

Skilful prescribing is essential. Always discuss and explain changes to the medication. Use a drug card for outpatient prescribing (*see Prescribing*). Review! Symptom control takes time. One intervention or change of medication is rarely enough. Review regularly and adjust medication (daily at first).

Attention to detail is essential. Small details about a dose or when an analgesic can safely be increased can (and often does) make the difference between a patient remaining comfortable at home and being admitted to hospital as an emergency.

The family must be included, as they are usually involved with organizing the complex regime of medication and because they are usually worried about the symptoms (especially new symptoms). Most symptoms are made worse by family tension and may only resolve when the family's emotional needs are addressed (*see Family support*). When carers are not supported home care often collapses unnecessarily.

Rehabilitation is usually possible once symptoms are controlled. Rehabilitation is often mental and emotional as much as physical. The control of symptoms releases a person to get back to more important issues, like the quality of their remaining life (*see Rehabilitation*).

Symptom control empowers a doctor to help, even though the patient is not curable. Patients hope for support rather than miracles. Listen and ask questions before giving explanation or reassurance, to avoid making incorrect assumptions. New symptoms can be frightening. A common fear is: "Does this mean the cancer is spreading?" Some symptoms have special significance for the patient. It can be important to ask, "Have you known anyone else with cancer?" which can bring fears to light (*see Counselling*).

Routine Measurements of temperature, pulse, respirations, and blood pressure are not necessary in inpatients where the aim is symptom control.

PATIENT ASSESSMENT

A full assessment of the patient's situation lays the foundation for a relationship of trust. It involves both the patient and the family. It involves gathering information, listing problems and planning for the future. It can be tiring for the patient and the information may need to be gathered over a period of time. The following information is usually relevant.

History of present illness:

- Presenting symptoms
- Surgery\RT\chemotherapy – consultant's names
- Nerve blocks
- What has been the worst part?

Past Medical History

Drugs:

- List (while discussing the bottles themselves)
- Analgesic history
- Steroid history
- Preferences\Allergies
- Write out a drug card (*see prescribing*)

Symptom list. The top 20 symptoms in this list should be enquired about in all patients.

Pain
Anorexia
Nausea
Vomiting
Sore mouth
Dysphagia
Constipation\Diarrhoea
Urinary problems
Dyspnoea
Cough
Weakness
Weight loss
pressure areas
Fluid retention
Drowsiness
Confusion
Insomnia
Anxiety
Depression

Bleeding
Paralysis
Itching
Jaundice
Hiccups
Sweating
Thirst
Fistula

Mobility\Self-care\Diet

Social history

- Occupational history
- Hobbies\Interests
- Home conditions (bed, toilet, stairs etc.)
- Responsibilities\Dependents
- Daily routine
- Carers\Helpers
- Finances\Will

Family history

- Genogram (family tree)
- Family feelings
- Deaths in the family (what, where, how)
- Insight of children
- Useful question: "Who is like who in your family?"

Spiritual aspects

- Do you have any church support?
- Do you have any faith or beliefs
- Is a minister\priest visiting?
- Do you have any ideas about why you became ill?

Examination

- oral thrush?
- skin nodules\enlarged nodes?
- oedema?
- neurological signs?
- chest – wheeze? effusion?
- liver metastases?
- faecal impaction?
- pressure sores?

N.B. An examination can be therapeutic of itself if unhurried. Touch is a powerful form of non-verbal communication.

Patients aims?

Problem list + Management plan for each problem

Any explanations given?

Others involved?

- GP
- District Nurse
- Consultant surgeon\oncologist
- Pain clinic
- Hospice consultant
- Macmillan nurse
- Marie Curie night sitters
- Physiotherapist
- Occupational therapist
- Social Worker
- Psychologist\Counsellor
- Care Assistants
- Warden
- Home help
- Meals on Wheels

A patient questionnaire can be a simple and effective method of assessing a patient's needs and concerns, and can reduce the strain of repeated assessments by different members of the team. Administration of the questionnaire can be therapeutic in itself, allowing patients to focus on areas of difficulty that they may not have addressed before. Patient's coping by denial may find it threatening and may refuse to co-operate, but most patients find it helpful. The MacAdam questionnaire, below, covers symptoms, spirits, knowledge and support, and has been shown to be effective in assessing areas of difficulty.

Reference:
Fowlie M, Berkeley J, Dingwall-Fordyce I. Quality of life in advanced cancer: the benefits of asking the patient. Palliative Medicine 1989; 3: 55-59.

PATIENT QUESTIONNAIRE TO ASSESS NEEDS

1. My appetite has been good

2. I have felt nauseated

3. I have had pain

4. I have found breathing easy

5. I have felt drowsy

6. I have been constipated

7. I have had diarrhoea

8. I have had worries about how my spouse or family will cope in the future

9. My beliefs and personal philosophy of life have helped me

10. I have adequate opportunities of expressing love and affection with my loved one or partner

11. My knowledge about my treatment and illness has been ...

12. I have been concerned about the results of my treatment (or investigation)

13. I have been looking forward to the future

14. I have felt life was worth living

15. I have felt down or low-spirited

16. I have felt afraid

17. The support I have had from my family and friends has been ...

18. I have felt needed by my family and friends

19. I have been able to share how I am feeling now with another person

20. Contacts outside my family e.g. church, club, work etc. have been ...

Reference:
MacAdam *et al*. Palliative Medicine 1987; 1: 37-47.

ABDOMINAL DISTENSION

Abdominal distension may be due to:

- Tumour masses
- Ascites
- Constipation
- Intestinal obstruction
- Malabsorbtion
- Steroids
- Lactulose
- Air swallowing (anxiety)

Ultrasound scan can be helpful in diagnosing the cause, and detecting tumour masses or ascites.

Steroids cause abdominal protrusion due to weakened abdominal muscles. Lactulose can cause excessive wind in some patients.

ADVANCED DIRECTIVES

An advanced directive ("living will") is a witnessed document stating a patient's wishes about medical care or life-prolonging treatment. Advanced directives are being increasingly used in the United States.

A proxy may be nominated to act as a sympathetic interpreter of the patient's wishes.

The purpose of advanced directives is to give patients the right to choose or refuse life-sustaining treatment in the event of them becoming incapable of stating their own wishes. The main intention is to protect individuals from inappropriately intensive treatments, such as the mechanical ventilation of patients with advanced motor neurone disease and respiratory failure.

The advantage of advanced directives is that they encourage communication and debate about the wishes of patients. The patient must have thought about their wishes in order to complete such a document. The problem is that patients with far-advanced disease may change their minds about what they imagined they would want when they were well.

Euthanasia is rightly illegal. Advanced directives cannot be used to request euthanasia. Patients have no rights to be killed and no rights to request to be killed. Such a right would place an unacceptable duty on doctors to kill patients, and would be a negative and destructive solution to the problems of suffering (*see Ethical issues*).

Reference:
Hope T. Advanced directives about medical treatment. Br Med J 1992; 304: 398

AIDS

AIDS means Acquired Immune Deficiency Syndrome. AIDS was first described in 1981. The virus, HIV type 3, was discovered in 1983. Since reporting of AIDS began in January 1982 there have been 8,425 AIDS cases (7% female) in the UK up to December 1993, of whom 64% have died. There were 176 new cases reported in November 1993. The probable route of transmission is homosexual in 75%, heterosexual in 10%, blood products in 6%, injecting drug abuse in 5% and mother to baby in 1%. There have been 19,524 reports of HIV infection since reports began in 1984 to August 1993.

The HIV virus is transmitted in blood products, by sexual intercourse or from mother to unborn child, and infects T4 lymphocytes (destroying the immune response) monocytes and brain cells.

Antibodies to the HIV virus are usually detectable within 1-2 months of infection. Seropositive individuals are symptomfree for many years, but most (and probably all) HIV positive individuals will progress to develop AIDS, and 50% within 10 years. The median time from infection to AIDS is 7-10 years.

CD4 count (T4 helper-lymphocyte count) below $0.35 \times 10^9 \backslash l$ indicates a high chance of developing AIDS, and is taken by some as an indication to start zidovudine treatment. A CD4 count that is rapidly falling indicates a poor prognosis.

HIV disease is classified into 4 stages:

1: A mononucleosis-like illness may occur 2-6 weeks after infection
2: Asymptomatic period (several years)
3: Persistent generalized lymphadenopathy
4: AIDS, characterized by:

- Weight loss, fevers, diarrhoea (4a)
- Neurological damage (4b)
- PCP and opportunistic infections (4c)
- KS and secondary cancers (4d).

PCP = Pneumocystis pneumonia
KS = Kaposi's Sarcoma
OI = Opportunistic infection

In the early stages of AIDS there is a good response to treatment and often full recovery of weight and energy levels. As the disease progresses, OIs recur, with a shortening interval between each episode of illness, and weight loss and fatigue become more marked, sometimes with behavioural and neurological changes. In the advanced phase there is increasing fatigue, infections are constant or worsening and there is often an element of dementia and sometimes blindness.

Median survival with AIDS depends on the pattern of the disease:

KS alone (31 months)
PCP alone (24 months)

KS with PCP or OIs (7 months)
Malignancy (4 months)
Severe dementia (2 months).

Symptom control generally follows the same principles as in cancer patients. 40 outpatients with AIDS (Welch, 1991) ranked their symptoms in order of distress as:

- Tiredness
- Poor appetite
- Troublesome skin
- Sleeplessness
- Sore mouth or throat
- Cough
- Weight loss
- Diarrhoea
- Sore or itchy bottom
- Chest problems
- Stuffy nose
- Fear
- Sore muscles
- Sweats
- Discomfort in hands\feet
- Headaches
- Changes in appearance
- Sore genitals
- Trouble swallowing
- Sore or gritty eyes

Antibiotics are still indicated in advanced AIDS to prevent the recurrence of opportunistic infections. Fluconazole and acyclovir should not be stopped until the final stages, when the patient is unable to swallow, because the recurrence of thrush or herpes will cause distress.

Daily IV ganciclovir can prevent the worsening of CMV retinitis (which can cause blindness) and it may occasionally be indicated even in advanced disease. If treatment is stopped the retinitis does not usually progress for 2-3 weeks, and a patient in the terminal phase who stops ganciclovir can be reassured that their sight will not suddenly deteriorate.

Zidovudine can be stopped, once the patient reaches the terminal phase of illness, but this implies acceptance of the terminal phase of disease However, there is no evidence of benefit from zidovudine, once the terminal stages are reached and 40% develop side-effects, (most commonly anaemia, but also nausea, myalgia, severe headache, or insomnia). Paracetamol, NSAIDs, and morphine can increase serum levels of zidovudine (by competing for hepatic glucuronidation) and increase toxicity.

Anti-tuberculous therapy for infection wih MAI (Mycobacterium avium intracellulare) can be stopped. In patients with abdominal pains and diarrhoea, steroids and NSAIDs provide more effective symptom control.

Steroids can be safely used in AIDS to improve appetite and well-being. The theoretical risk of accelerating OIs is not in fact a problem, and steroids, (dexamethasone 2-4mg a day) can dramatically improve symptoms such as sweating, fevers, musculoskeletal pain, neuropathic pain and headache or vomiting due to raised ICP.

There is a small risk of rapid progression of KS lesions, in which case steroids may need to be stopped. KS lesions in the oropharynx or anogenital regions may therefore preclude the use of steroids, since any worsening of the lesions could cause distressing discomfort.

Common problems in advanced AIDS:

- KS
- Chronic pain
- Oesophagitis
- Proctitis
- Diarrhoea
- Skin problems
- Dementia
- Psychiatric features

KS (Kaposi's sarcoma) is a vascular tumour of endothelium that can affect any site. Pigmented red-blue lesions often first appear on the face, mouth or sole of the foot. Facial swelling due to lymphoedema can occur. Cosmetic treatment to the skin may require surgery, laser or intralesional chemotherapy. Bowel KS may cause bleeding or obstruction. Pulmonary KS may cause dyspnoea, wheeze or cough and sometimes pleural effusions. Chemotherapy is of no proven value and treatment is symtomatic. Chemotherapy can produce a response in 25-75% using a single agent (vincristine or etoposide) but prognosis is not improved. Radiotherapy can produce substantial regression of lesions, and may be useful for KS in:

- Oropharynx
- Larynx (hoarseness, stridor)
- Skin (for painful lesions)
- Facial lymphoedema

Steroids may occasionally cause rapid enlargement of KS lesions, and should be used with caution if there are KS lesions in delicate areas.

Chronic pain in AIDS occurs in 50% and is most commonly due to peripheral neuropathy, but visceral and soft tissue pains can occur (abdominal chest, retro-sternal, oropharygeal) due to KS or lymphoma. Other pains include:

- Headaches
- Skin pain
- Ano-rectal pain
- Joint pain
- Pressure sores
- Post-herpetic neuralgias
- Total body pain

Oesophagitis is common in AIDS and usually due to <u>Candida</u>. It can cause retrosternal pains (stabbing or burning), pharyngeal pain or dysphagia. Much less commonly it can be due to <u>Herpes simplex or CMV</u>. Treat with antacids or H2 antagonists, and candidal prophylaxis, (ketoconazole 400-800mg a day, fluconazole 100-400mg a day). The pain responds to paracetamol, NSAIDs or morphine. If symptoms persist prescribe oral acyclovir, 200-400mg 4 hourly, and consider endoscopy in a fit patient. A nasogastric tube may be necessary, either temporarily, awaiting a response, or permanently if this is the only means of relief.

Proctitis is common in AIDS and presents as pain, mucopurulent discharge or diarrhoea due to infection, inflammatory strictures, ulcers, fissures, warts, haemorrhoids or malignancy (lymphoma, KS, squamous carcinoma). Repeated cultures and biopsies often fail to demonstrate a cause. In a hospice setting it can be reasonable to treat with a combination of acyclovir, 200-400mg 4 hourly, (Herpes), amoxycillin (Gonococcus) and tetracycline (Chlamydia). Rarely, IV ganciclovir may be indicated for a recurrence of biopsy proven CMV. Pain relief, and stool softeners are essential, and other options may include radiotherapy for malignant lesions, colostomy or nerve blocks.

Diarrhoea occurs in 50% of patients with AIDS and may be due to faecal impaction or infection. Stool cultures may be necessary for a new episode, to isolate treatable pathogens: Salmonella, Shigella, Campylobacter, Clostridium difficile, Giardia and Isosporella belli. Infective patients (with salmonella or shigella) will need isolating. A combination of loperamide 1-4 capsules 6 hourly, and codeine phosphate, 30-90mg 4 hourly, is usually effective in controlling diarrhoea. For uncontrolled diarrhoea it may be appropriate to treat empirically with antibiotics and anti-parasite therapy (sulphonamides, quinolones, tetracyclines or metronidazole). The advice of an AIDS specialist and\or bacteriologist should be sought. <u>Octreotide</u> may control severe diarrhoea unresponsive to other measures (*see Diarrhoea*).

Skin problems in AIDS are very common and include fungal infections, eczema, psoriasis, folliculitis, Herpes simplex, Herpes zoster, molluscum contagiosum and scabies. <u>Scabies</u> should always be suspected if there is an atypical rash with crusting or nodules. It is highly contagious in AIDS because of the large numbers of mites. A dermatologist should be consulted. It is diagnosed on skin scrapings and treated with repeated applications of gamma benzene hexachloride.

Dementia is common in AIDS and occurs due to direct infection of brain cells with the HIV virus. It is detectable in 90% of patients with sensitive psychometric tests. Early changes include forgetfulness, poor concentration, apathy, irritability and slow speech. Progressive dementia, requiring institutional care, occurs in around 15%. The survival of patients with severe dementia is short (range 1-6 months, median 1.8 months), and therefore patients with AIDS-dementia may well be suitable for hospice programmes. Neurological features include ataxia, leg weakness with hyperreflexia, impaired eye movements, dysarthria and incontinence. The dementia progresses to global cognitive dysfunction and verbal and motor slowing to an akinetic state, with the patient lying awake but motionless, quietly confused and indifferent to their surroundings.

Psychiatric features of AIDS include Mood changes (anxiety, depression), psychotic features in 15% (hallucinations, delusions), and acute confusion. If there are sudden psychiatric changes, it may be appropriate to investigate, to exclude treatable CNS infections (CT scan for toxoplasmosis and lumbar puncture for crytococcus), and infections in chest or GI tract may need to be excluded in a toxic delerium. The CT scan in dementia shows cerebral atrophy and ventricular dilatation. Most patients will be best managed with routine supportive measures, including psychotherapy and psychotropic drugs.

Further reading:
Sims R, Moss V, Terminal Care for People with AIDS, Edward Arnold, 1991.
Cole RM, Medical Aspects of Care for the person with AIDS: a palliative care prespective, Palliative Medicine, 1991; 5: 96-111
Welch JM *et al*. Symptoms of HIV disease, Palliative Medicine 1991; 5: 46-51.

ALCOHOL

Alcohol is probably the most ancient medicine, and still has a place in palliative care. There are 5 types of alcoholic beverage: beer, wine, sherry, liqueurs and spirits.

Many hospices have a drinks trolley that follows the drug trolley on its evening rounds. There are no randomized hospice studies, as yet, on the effects of alcohol, but a study in a geriatric hospital showed that the introduction of alcohol had beneficial psycho-social effects, improved group morale, reduced irritability and worry, and sometimes improved sleep patterns, alertness, self-care and functional status.

The pharmacological effects of alcohol include:

- Appetite stimulation
- Increased gastro-intestinal secretions
- Mild sedation
- Euphoria (low doses)
- Relaxation (low doses)
- Analgesia
- Diuresis
- Skin vasodilation

Contra-indications to the use of alcohol are:

- History of alcoholism
- Alcohol intolerance
- Gastric ulcer
- Potential drug interactions

Note that alcohol causes no ill effects in patients with liver disease or liver metastases. A history of alcoholism – even years ago, is an absolute contra-indication to alcohol. Alcohol intolerance can occur as a paraneoplastic syndrome. Tumour pain induced by even small doses of alcohol is well described in Hodkin's disease, but also occurs in other tumours, especially cancers of the cervix, bladder and lung.

Drug interactions with alcohol include:

- Disulfiram-like reaction
- Excess sedation with morphine and psychotropics
- Inhibition of drug metabolism (tricyclics)

Alcohol may cause a disulfiram-like reaction (headache, flushing, nausea, palpitations) in some patients on metronidazole, and less commonly chloramphenicol, oral sulphonylureas and some cephalosporin antibiotics.

Alcohol withdrawal, in a patient accustomed to regular alcohol intake, can cause delerium tremens, which may not develop for several days, usually after 1-3 days, with:

- Tremor
- Fever, sweats, tachycardia
- Agitation
- Hallucinations – visual
- Siezures (generalized not focal)

Heminevrin (Chlormethiazole) is the treatment of choice to manage the withdrawal phase, (although giving the patient alcohol will reduce symptoms for a time). Heminevrin is a powerful sedative, anti-convulsant and anxiolytic. A suitable heminevrin regime might be:

- 3 capsules QID for 3 days
- 2 capsules QID for 3 days
- 1 capsules QID for 3 days

Further reading:
Kerr D. Alcohol and palliative care. Palliative Medicine 1992; 6: 185-201.

ANAEMIA

Anaemia can be defined as an Hb level below 8g\dl. The common causes of anaemia are:

- Chronic disease (normocytic)
- Iron deficiency from chronic bleeding (microcytic)
- Marrow invasion (leuco-erythroblastic)

Patients with marrow invasion from solid tumours tend to have a prognosis of only a few weeks.

Symptoms of anaemia include:

- Dizziness
- Palpitations
- Angina
- Dyspnoea
- Fatigue

Anaemia of gradual onset may be symptomless.

Active bleeding in advanced disease is not an indication for transfusion (unless the bleeding has been controlled) because transfusion simply worsens the bleeding. Bleeding tends to slow down and stop as the Hb level falls, and a transfusion may simply re-start the bleeding, which often causes more distress than the anaemia.

The indications for a blood transfusion are symptoms due to anaemia, but not asymptomatic anaemia. Anaemia of gradual onset, with Hb levels around 7g\l, can be asymptomatic in patients who are leading a quiet existence. Weakness and fatigue are often due to the advanced malignant disease, rather than the anaemia, and transfusion may only give a boost for 1-2 days (which may still be worthwhile for special events, such as attending a wedding). A trial of blood transfusion may be indicated for some patients, and if it makes them feel better it can be repeated. Stored blood can drop its pH, which makes it give up oxygen less easily, and optimum oxygen carriage may not occur for 72 hours after transfusion.

The technique of blood transfusion involves:

- Start an infusion of normal saline
- Give packed cells
- Allow 4 hours per unit
- Consider frusemide, 20mg per unit
- Monitor pulse and temperature

Repeated transfusions for chronic anaemia can become inappropriate. Stopping the transfusions does not necessarily lead to death. The patient may live for some time, with a very low Hb level, and may prefer this to the nuisance of repeated transfusions.

Iron therapy may be indicated for a patient with a reasonably long prognosis, if bleeding has caused an iron deficiency anaemia (MCV below 76 fl). Oral iron stains the motions black. The Hb level should rise at the rate of about 1g per week, provided the marrow is normal and there is no continued bleeding. Ferrous sulphate, 200mg TID, is the first choice preparation. If side-effects occur (constipation, or occasionally diarrhoea and nausea) then lower the dose or change to Ferrous gluconate, 300-600mg TID. Iron absorbtion is probably very poor from the slow-release preparations, which should be avoided. Vitamin C can increase the absorbtion or oral iron.

Vitamin B12 I.M. Hydroxycobalamin, 1mg\ml, is given monthly following gastrectomy or resection of the terminal ileum to prevent megaloblastic anaemia (MCV above 96 fl), which can develop after liver stores of B12 are exhausted (which normally takes several years).

Epoetin is genetically engineered human erythropoetin, the hormone synthesised by the kidneys that controls red cell production. There are 2 preparations:

- epoetin alfa (Eprex)
- epoetin beta (Recormon)

Epoetin is licensed for use to treat the anaemia of chronic renal failure and greatly reduces the need for repeated transfusions. It is given by weekly SC injection to achieve a monthly rise in Hb of around 1g\dl, after which a lower dose is given weekly as maintainance therapy. The main side-effect is hypertension. It has been used experimentally in cancer patients with marrow involvement and in the anaemia of myeloma and it may come to have a place in the management of some cancer patients or AIDS anaemia due to zidovudine.

Reference:
Oster W, Hermann F, Gamm H *et al*. Erythropoetin for the treatment of anaemia of malignancy associated with neoplastic bone marrow infiltration. J Clin Oncol 1990; 8: 956-62.

ANALGESICS

Analgesics are drugs that reduce the ability to feel pain. Their main side-effect is constipation. Co-analgesics can control certain types of pain, but are not normally classified as analgesics. They include NSAIDs, tricyclics, anti-convulsants, steroids, anxiolytics and antibiotics (*see Pain*).

CLASSIFICATION OF ANALGESICS

Mild Analgesics (Non-opioid)

- Paracetamol
- Aspirin

Medium-Strength Opioids

- Codeine
- Dihydrocodeine
- Dextropropoxyphene

Strong Opioids

- Morphine
- MST
- Diamorphine

Agonist\Antagonists Opioids

- Buprenorphine
- Meptazinol
- Nalbuphine

Alternative Strong Opioids

- Oxycodone
- Methadone
- Dextromoramide
- Phenazocine

Paracetamol, 1gm 4 hourly, will control mild visceral pain. It is available as 500mg suppositories. If morphine is given too early, for mild pains, it can cause excessive sedation and puts the patient off using morphine altogether. Apply the analgesic ladder:

Mild pain – Paracetamol
Moderate pain – Co-proxamol
Severe pain – Morphine

Medium-strength opioids include codeine, dihydrocodeine and dextropropoxyphene. Co-proxamol, 2 tablets, 4 hourly, is the moderate opioid of choice. Each tablet contains dextropropoxyphene 32.5mg and paracetamol 325mg. It is less constipating than codeine. If the effect of 2 co-proxamol, 4 hourly, is partial or does not last the full 4 hours, then morphine is indicated, starting at 5mg-10mg morphine 4 hourly, and increasing every 4 hours until pain-free. (See Morphine). Codeine and dihydrocodeine, 60mg 4 hourly, are both equi-analgesic with 2 co-proxamol tablets, but tend to be very constipating. DHC Continus, 60mg BD, is slow release dihydrocodeine, and has the advantage of a twice daily dosage. Combined analgesics, except Tylex and Solpadol, all contain low doses of codeine (or dihydrocodeine) and are therefore weak analgesics (see table).

COMBINED ANALGESICS

	Codeine	Paracetamol	Aspirin
co-codamol	8mg	500mg	–
co-dydramol	10mg*	500mg	–
co-codaprin	8mg	–	400mg
Solpadeine	8mg	500mg	–
Tylex	30mg	500mg	–
Solpadol	30mg	500mg	–

*Dihydrocodeine

Morphine is the drug of choice for continuous cancer pain. If pain is only partly controlled by 4 hourly co-proxamol, start oral morphine in a dose of 5-10mg 4 hourly. Morphine, MST and diamorphine injections are discussed separately (*see Diamorphine, Morphine*).

Agonist-antagonist drugs are of 2 types: nalorphine-like and buprenorphine-like.

Nalorphine was recognized in 1956 as having a double action. In lower doses it antagonizes morphine, yet at higher doses it has analgesic activity at the kappa receptor. Pentazocine (Fortral) is a nalorphine-like drug, but also acts at other receptors (sigma) and has unpleasant side-effects.

Buprenorphine is a partial agonist at the mu receptor. It is also an antagonist because it has a very high affinity for the mu receptor and blocks the action of morphine at the same receptors. A partial agonist has less effect at the receptor than a complete agonist such as morphine, and therefore has a ceiling effect, meaning that above a certain dose no further analgesia is achieved. Meptazinol (Meptid) is a buprenorphine-like drug but has no advantages over buprenorphine.

OPIOID RECEPTORS

	mu receptor	kappa receptor
Morphine	+	
Nalorphine	–	+
Buprenorphine	p+	

Strong opioid alternatives to morphine are only occasionally needed. If a patient develops side-effects with one opioid drug, they may still tolerate another. There is no known analgesic superior to morphine, and other analgesics are usually best avoided, but about 2% of patients cannot tolerate morphine because of severe nausea, uncontrollable with anti-emetics. The following opioids can be useful for the few patients who cannot tolerate morphine, or in special circumstances.

- Buprenorphine
- Dextromoramide
- Methadone
- Phenazocine
- Oxycodone

Buprenorphine (Temgesic) is a useful alternative to morphine in the lower dose range. It is effective orally or sublingually (useful in dysphagia). Each dose lasts 6-9 hours. It is available as 0.2mg and 0.4mg tablets. It is almost as effective sublingually as by injection, so there is very little place for the injection.

EQUI-ANALGESIC DOSES	
Sublingual Buprenorphine (6-8 hourly)	Oral Morphine (4 hourly)
0.2mg	10mg
0.4mg	20mg
0.6mg	30mg

Buprenorphine is only licensed for use up to 0.4mg 8 hourly, but some patients may take higher doses. It is limited by a "ceiling effect" – increasing the dose above 0.8mg 8 hourly does not increase the analgesic effect, but can increase the side-effects (nausea, dizziness). It is not as effective as morphine for controlling dyspnoea. Buprenorphine is a "partial agonist". It binds more avidly than morphine to the opioid receptors, but is less powerful in its analgesic effect. This is not clinically important when changing to morphine – an oral dose of morphine still acts within 1 hour, even if the patient has recently taken buprenorphine, (because there are still enough spare receptors for the morphine molecules). Where the interaction with morphine is clinically important is in patients on higher doses of morphine (above 60mg 4 hourly) when the erroneous addition of buprenorphine can cause pain, (because it binds more avidly to opioid receptors, displacing the morphine molecules).

Dextromoramide (Palfium), 5mg tablet, is a powerful short-acting analgesic. It is effective sublingually, and can be very useful for patients with severe pain on swallowing. 2.5-5mg is taken sublingually, about 1 hour before eating. It can also be helpful before painful dressings, and there is also a 10mg suppository.

Methadone (Physeptone), is available as a cough linctus (2mg in 5ml) and as a mixture (5mg in 5ml). It is mainly used to suppress an irritating cough, and sometimes seems to be helpful even in patients already taking morphine. It is well-absorbed and slowly metabolized, and therefore it has a long half-life of 15 hours after a single dose (compared to 2 hours for oral morphine), and it accumulates, which means that plasma levels go on increasing for several days if it is taken regularly. Therefore it can be difficult to titrate the dose to the level of pain, and severe drowsiness can develop 2-3 weeks after it is started, even if the dose has not been increased. It can be a useful alternative analgesic for patients who cannot tolerate morphine, and like morphine it has the advantage that it has a very high ceiling, so that the dose can be increased to high levels for severe pain if necessary. It should be given 6 hourly for the first 2 days, and then 8-12 hourly, and the patient must be warned about possible drowsiness.

Phenazacine (Narphen), 5mg tablet, is a powerful analgesic, and occasionally useful as an alternative to morphine. It is can be taken orally or sublingually, and is effective for 6 hours. Like most opioids it has a bitter taste. It has a "ceiling effect", and above 30mg 6 hourly, there is no further increase in analgesic effect. Side-effects include nausea and dizziness.

EQUI-ANALGESIC DOSES	
Phenazocine (6 hourly)	Morphine (4 hourly)
2.5mg	10mg
5mg	20mg
10mg	40mg
20mg	80mg
30mg	120mg

Oxycodone pectinate (Proladone) suppositories, 30mg, have a duration of action of 8 hours, and can be useful for some patients who cannot tolerate morphine. They are available by special order from Boots. They are equi-analgesic with oral morphine, e.g. a patient who is pain controlled on 30mg oral morphine 4 hourly will be pain controlled on 60mg oxycodone 8 hourly. It is possible to use 3 or 4 suppositories at a time if necessary. (Palliative Medicine 1992; 6: 79)

Equi-analgesic doses of the commonly used analgesics need to be known, when changing from one analgesic to another, so that the patient does not lose confidence in the new analgesic due to pain breakthrough (too little opioid) or excessive sedation (too much opioid). Changing from medium-strength opioids to morphine is needed as cancer pain increases. The table below shows that the equivalent dose is 5mg of morphine 4 hourly, but the starting dose is usually 10mg if the reason for changing is increasing pain.

EQUI-ANALGESIC DOSES		4 hourly Oral Morphine
Co-proxamol	2 tabs	5mg
Codeine	60mg	5mg
Dihydrocodeine	60mg	5mg

Strong alternatives to morphine are occasionally needed for special circumstances, most commonly morphine-induced vomiting. For example a patient on 20mg of morphine every 4 hours will need 5mg phenazocine every 6 hours for an equivalent analgesic effect. More commonly, patients who have been started on these alternatives are changed to morphine. A patient who is pain-controlled on dextromoramide 15mg every 2 or 3 hours, will require 45mg morphine every 4 hours for an equivalent effect. If any opioid has helped for any length of time, then it is likely that the patient will be painfree on the correct dose of 4 hourly morphine. Note that the duration of action of the analgesic drugs varies, with dextromoramide lasting about 2-3 hours, morphine 4 hours and most of the others 6-8 hours.

The table below is a guide, and applies to ORAL analgesics when taken regularly, for the control of a pain that is opioid-responsive.

EQUI-ANALGESIC DOSE TABLE FOR STRONG OPIOIDS		Oral morphine 4 hourly
Buprenorphine (Temgesic)	0.2mg	10mg
Methadone (Physeptone)	5mg	10mg
Dextromoramide (Palfium)	5mg	15mg
Oxycodone (Proladone)	30mg PR	15mg
Phenazocine (Narphen)	5mg	20mg

Other alternatives to morphine should be avoided in the control of cancer pain. No analgesic is superior to morphine. In particular pentazocine (Fortral) causes unpleasant mental effects, Diconal (dipipanone 10mg is combined with 30mg of cyclizine) causes too much sedation, and pethidine is a weak analgesic orally that only lasts 2-3 hours and in higher doses produces toxic levels of its metabolite norpethidine that can cause twitching and convulsions.

Short-term pain control, such as is needed for changing painful dressings, includes:

- Sublingual dextromoramide (Palfium)
- Entonox
- IV alfentanil

Alfentanil (Rapifen) is an ultra-short acting opioid, normally used in anaesthetics, which may occasionally be useful to control severe incident pain, such as pain on changing a dressing or being moved to a different bed. The dose is 500 micrograms IV over 30 seconds, which is very unlikely to cause any respiratory depression in a patient already on morphine. Doxapram (Dopram) a respiratory stimulant, should be available. 50mg of doxapram IV over 30 seconds will reverse any respiratory depression without causing pain breakthrough, and is therefore preferred to naloxone.

Reference:
Hanks GW, Hoskin PJ. Opioid analgesics in the management of pain in patients with cancer. A review. Palliative Medicine 1987; 1: 1-25.

ANOREXIA

Anorexia means loss of appetite. It occurs in about 70% of patients with advanced cancer (possibly due to tumour peptides). Often no specific cause can be found, but the following should be excluded:

- Oral thrush
- Nausea
- Constipation
- Anxiety or depression
- Drugs (cytotoxics, digoxin, NSAIDs)

Anxiety is a common factor in anorexia. Patients in the secure environment of a hospice often start to eat better.

Dexamethasone, 4mg daily, improves the appetite in 80% usually for several weeks (although a placebo will help 50%). Side effects can be a problem (*see Steroids*).

Progestagens such as medroxyprogesterone acetate or megestrol acetate may improve appetite, and may be an alternative to steroids for some patients. There is no evidence that other drugs such as cyproheptadine improve appetite. Vitamin C, 500mg QID for 4-6 weeks, may improve appetite.

Metoclopramide (Maxolon) 10-20mg before meals can help, if poor appetite is due to a feeling of fullness or heartburn (small stomach syndrome).

A dietician can give helpful advice. Simple things can make all the difference, e.g. large helpings can be demoralizing, whereas smaller portions can actually improve appetite. A range of supplementary foods are available. (*see Diet*).

Explanation helps: the body needs less food when inactive and ill. It may be easier to eat little and often, rather than at set meal times. No foods are harmful. Taste changes are common and new tastes may be preferred. Feeding does not prolong life, and can become a burden.

Intensive feeding via a nasogastric tube, or via the IV route, does not improve appetite, weight, well-being or prognosis and has no place in the management of anorexia.

ANTIBIOTICS

Infections should be treated if they are causing distressing symptoms, regardless of prognosis. Specimens should be sent for sensitivity tests whenever possible.

Narrow-spectrum antibiotics are used to treat specific problems. Penicillin is used to treat Streptococcal infections, and is also active against some Gram positive anaerobes. Skin infections are often due to Staph. aureus and usually respond to flucloxacillin (and occasionally to co-trimoxozole). Patients allergic to penicillin can be treated with erythromycin (although this often causes abdominal discomfort and diarrhoea). Urinary infections are usually due to E. coli or other Gram negative bacilli, and narrow spectrum antibiotics may be the most appropriate treatment once the results of sensitivity tests are available. Metronidazole is very useful to treat anaerobic organisms causing smell (*see Smell*). Narrow spectrum antibiotics include:

NARROW SPECTRUM ANTIBIOTICS				
	Gram Pos	Staph aureus	Gram Neg	Anaerobes
Penicillin	+			(+)
Flucloxacillin		+		
Erythromycin	+	+		(+)
Trimethoprim (Ipral)			+	
Pivmecillinam (Selexid)			+	
Nitrofurantoin (Furadantin)	(+)		+	
Metronidazole				+

Broad-spectrum antibiotics are active against a wide range of both Gram positive and Gram negative organisms. They are very useful in the initial treatment of urinary and chest infections, before the results of sensitivity tests are available. Some broad spectrum antibiotics, such as tetracycline, are less valuable because many strains of Streptococci and Staph. aureus are now resistant. In persistent infections, the infecting organisms can develop resistance, and choice of antibiotic should be guided by repeat sensitivity tests. Cephalexin is active against most Gram positive organisms, but not the Strep. faecalis group. Ciprofloxacin is reserved for infections resistant to other antibiotics, but has a variable action against Gram positive organisms and Staph. aureus. Co-amoxiclav (Augmentin) and chloramphenicol are both very broad spectrum, and are also active against anaerobes, and are useful alternatives to metronidazole if the patient cannot tolerate it. Chloramphenicol is a useful antibiotic for resistant infections in terminal care, and has a very low incidence of side-effects (and marrow toxicity occurs in only 1 in 30,000, which is an acceptable risk in this situation).

BROAD SPECTRUM ANTIBIOTICS

	Gram Pos	Staph aureus	Gram Neg	Anaerobes
Amoxycillin	+		+	
Cephalexin (Keflex)	+		+	
Co-trimoxazole (Septrin)	+	(+)	+	
Ciprofloxacin (Ciproxin)	+	(+)	+	
Co-amoxiclav(Augmentin)	+	+	+	+
Chloramphenicol	+	+	+	+

ANTI-EMETICS

Anti-emetics are drugs that reduce nausea and vomiting.
They can be classified by site of action (see Table):

CLASSIFICATION OF ANTI-EMETICS BY SITE OF ACTION

Site	Anti-emetic
The Vomiting Centre: (Anti-cholinergic\Anti-histamines)	Cyclizine Promethazine
The CTZ: (Dopamine antagonists)	Haloperidol Chlorpromazine
The GI tract (gastro-kinetic)	Metoclopramide* Domperidone
The Cortex	Lorazepam Cannabinoids
5HT3 receptor antagonists	Ondansetron Metoclopramide*

* Metoclopramide acts peripherally on the gut and on the CTZ centrally, and in high doses (100-200mg per day) also acts at the 5HT3 receptors.

What is the CTZ? CTZ means chemoreceptor trigger zone, which is a group of neurones in the medulla, close to another group which forms the vomiting centre. In 1951 it was noted that ablation of the CTZ in the cat abolished apomorphine-induced vomiting (and also vomiting due to other blood-bourne chemical emetics) but left intact the vomiting caused by intragastric copper sulphate. Thus 2 mechanisms were suggested. Drugs and toxins seemed to act via the CTZ, where there is a concentration of dopamine receptors in animal studies, whereas direct gastric causes act directly on the vomiting centre, where there is a concentration of histamine receptors. However, the neurophysiology is complex and has been mainly studied in the cat, and may be different in man.

GUIDE TO ANTI-EMETIC POTENCY AND SITE OF ACTION

Anti-emetic	CTZ	Vomiting Centre	5HT3
Hyoscine		++	
Cyclizine		+++	
Domperidone	+\-		
Metoclopramide	+		+ (high dose)
Prochlorperazine	++		
Chlorpromazine	++	+	
Haloperidol	+++		
Methotrimeprazine	+++	++	
Ondansetron			++

Useful anti-emetics in palliative care include:

- Cyclizine
- Metoclopramide
- Haloperidol
- Methotrimeprazine
- Ondansetron

Cyclizine (Valoid) 50mg 6 hourly, orally, IM, suppository or by SC infusion, is an anti-histamine and anti-cholinergic and acts at the cholinergic receptors of the vomiting centre. It is a very useful general purpose anti-emetic, especially indicated for N and V due to intestinal causes, raised intracranial pressure, or motion sickness. The suppositories need to be specially made up. The main side-effect is a dry mouth.

Metoclopramide (Maxalon), 10-20mg 6 hourly, or 60-80mg by SC infusion, acts as a dopamine antagonist at the CTZ and also at 5HT3 receptors in the gut wall. It is also gastro-kinetic, increasing gastric and gut motility and encouraging stomach emptying. It is used in the Squashed Stomach Syndrome, to reduce heartburn, nausea, fullness, wind or hiccups, and is a first-line drug (with haloperidol) for opioid-induced vomiting and is used in high doses as an anti-emetic during chemotherapy. It has been used in very high doses (240mg per day) to overcome gastric stasis. It has the particular advantage of causing very little drowsiness. There is a risk of extra-pyramidal side-effects, and it should never be given to young female patients because there is a high risk of a severe reaction (oculo-gyric crisis, requiring IV benztropine 1mg to reverse the effect).

Haloperidol (Serenace), 1.5-2.5mg orally 12 hourly or subcutaneously, 5-10mg per 24 hours, is a powerful anti-emetic that acts by blocking the dopamine receptors in the CTZ. It is a first-line anti-emetic for non-specific "tumour load" nausea or vomiting, or opioid-induced or uraemic vomiting. It causes no anti-cholinergic side-effects but does cause extra-pyramidal effects in some patients, starting with stiffness of the hands (e.g. difficulty knitting) or eye muscles (difficulty moving the eyes across the page when reading) which can progess to a Parkinsonian picture with rigidity and bradykinesia. These effects can sometimes be reduced with benzhexol (Artane) starting with 1mg daily and increasing gradually to 1mg 6 hourly.

Methotrimeprazine (Nozinan) is available orally as 25mg tablets, 25-50mg 6-8 hourly, or injection (25mg\ml) for IM or SC infusion, 25-200mg per 24 hours. is related to chlorpromazine but is a more powerful anti-emetic and has the advantage that it can be used subcutaneously. It is indicated for severe nausea or vomiting that is resistant to other anti-emetics. It can be combined with diamorphine and dexamethasone and Buscopan for subcutaneous infusion. It is very sedating and causes a dry mouth and in patients over 50 it can cause marked postural hypotension, (warn ambulatory patients).

Ondansetron (Zofran) 8mg 8-12 hourly acts as an antagonist in the gut at the serotonin 5HT3 receptors. It is currently reserved for the control of chemotherapy or radiotherapy induced vomiting, but may come to have a wider application in palliative medicine. Ondansetron selectively blocks only the 5HT3 receptors, and is more effective for chemotherapy-induced nausea than high dose metoclopramide. The dose of ondansetron is 8mg IV and then 8mg orally BD for 5 days, to prevent late nausea. Ondansetron is potentiated by dexamethasone 20mg IV then 4mg daily.

Chemotherapy-induced vomiting is particularly severe with cisplatinum, and also associated especially with dacarbazine, cyclophosphamide, lomustine and doxorubicin. It is probably due to release of 5HT from the gut, which stimulates the CTZ in the medulla. With cisplatinum, the combination of metoclopramide, dexamethasone and midazolam prevents nausea in 60%. High-dose metoclopramide (200mg IV) blocks 5HT type 3 receptors, as well as dopamine receptors.

Subcutaneous infusions of anti-emetics are particularly useful to gain control of nausea or vomiting or for the longterm management of malignant intestinal obstruction. The following drugs are commonly used (*see also Subcutaneous infusions*):

ANTI-EMETICS FOR SUBCUTANEOUS INFUSIONS	
	Usual starting dose per 24 hours
● Cyclizine	50mg
● Metoclopramide	60mg
● Haloperidol	5mg
● Methotrimeprazine	75mg

Suppositories can be useful in the home to control mild nausea and vomiting before reverting to oral anti-emetics to maintain control. Some patients prefer suppositories to tablets or an infusion and some do not. The following are used:

- ● Prochlorperazine
- ● Domperidone
- ● Cyclizine

Prochlorperazine (Stemetil), 25mg 8 hourly, is useful and causes little sedation. Domperidone (Motilium), 30-60mg 6 hourly is only a moderate strength anti-emetic, acting mainly peripherally, and will not control severe nausea. Cyclizine (Valoid), 50mg 6-8 hourly, may be more effective for nausea and vomiting due to gut causes, and the suppositories can be specially made up. Thiethylperazine (Torecan) 6.5mg 12 hourly is unfortunately no longer available as a suppository. It is a phenothiazine, and a powerful anti-emetic causing little sedation.

Other anti-emetics include chlorpromazine (Largactil), 10-25mg 6 hourly, which can be useful if sedation is needed as well as a mild anti-emetic. Buccastem, 3mg 12 hourly, is a buccal tablet of prochlorperazine (Stemetil) that is placed between the to p lip and the gum and left to dissolve. Cinnarizine (Stugeron) 15-30mg 8 hourly is an anti-histamine that causes little sedation, and can be particularly useful for nausea due to vertigo. Scopaderm TTS is a self-adhesive patch that releases 0.5mg of hyoscine hydrobromide over 72 hours. It is used to prevent travel sickness, but the plasma levels are usually too low to control established nausea or vomiting. Cisapride (Prepulsid) 10mg QID, increases gastric emptying but has no central anti-emetic action. It is effective for oesophageal reflux, but is expensive and has no advantage over metoclopramide.

ANXIETY

Anxiety means a state of apprehension or fear. Several studies have shown that 25% of cancer patients have significant anxiety or depression, or both.

Anxiety can be usefully classified into:

- Longstanding
- Episodic (part of an adjustment reaction)
- Situational (e.g. separation)
- Denial-related
- Severe (disturbing sleep, panic attacks)

Assessment of anxiety: The following questions are helpful:

1. Is it long-standing?
2. When and where does it occur?
3. Is there a specific worry or fear?
4. What is the patient's understanding of their illness? (Denial)
5. Is it affecting sleep or concentration?
6. Are there any physical symptoms:

- Sweating
- Tremor
- Palpitations

7. Have panic attacks occured?

Long-standing anxiety that is a personality trait will be difficult to alter. Ask the relatives. When or where anxiety occurs can reveal a pattern. It may be a separation anxiety, when their partner is away, or it may be worsened by relatives visiting. Anxiety about being left alone can get labelled as "attention seeking" – attention seeking patients require attention. Specific fears are usually amenable to counselling. Does the anxiety relate to a new symptom? ("Is the cancer spreading?"). Does it relate to weakness and fear of dependency? To beliefs about cancer? Has the patient known anyone else with cancer? Is it a fear about some aspect of dying? Discussing fears is helpful because resouces come to light (both internal and external) which re-frame the worry into a more manageable thought. It can be helpful to invite the patient to consider the thing they most fear. Nightmares are an expression of fear and it is always helpful to encourage patients to relate their nightmares which is a simple way of encouraging them to share and "externalize" their fears. Panic attacks are extremely frightening and if frequent or severe should be considered a medical emergency.

Management options in anxiety include:

- Medication
- Counselling
- Relaxation\Massage
- Family Meeting
- Psychologist

Medication may be needed for severe anxiety if it is affecting sleep or concentration or causing panic attacks or if there is an element of depression or paranoia. The following drugs can be helpful:

- Temazepam

- Amitriptyline
- Lorazepam
- Diazepam
- Haloperidol
- Propranolol

Temazepam, 10-60mg at night, is helpful if insomnia is the main problem.

Amitriptyline 25-75mg at night, may be more suitable if there is an element of depression.

Lorazepam 0.5-1mg 12 hourly, is useful for day-time anxiety, and is shorter-acting (half-life 12 hours) than diazepam (half-life 40 hours). It can be used sublingually for a rapoid effect.

Diazepam, 2-10mg at night, may be more useful if there is also a need for muscle relaxation.

Haloperidol 0.5-3mg 12 hourly, is helpful if there is an element of paranoia.

Propranolol 10-40mg 6 hourly, can be used to control the physical effects of anxiety (tremor, sweating, palpitations). When these are marked remember that thyrotoxicosis can (rarely) mimic anxiety.

HALF-LIVES OF ANXIOLYTIC BENZODIAZEPINES:	
	Half-life in hours
Diazepam	21-46
Clobezam	9-30
Lorazepam (Ativan)	8-25
Oxazepam	5-15
Medazepam (Nobrium)	1-7

Shorter-acting benzodiazepines are more suitable in patients with liver disease, although longterm use is more likely to cause withdrawal effects if they are stopped. Alprazolam, bromazepam and chlordiazepoxide (Librium) all have similar half-lives to lorazepam.

Counselling: Most anxiety responds to listening and support. The person has to find new ways of thinking about their life and future. All their assumptions (their "assumptive world") have to change. It can be very helpful to explain this and to reframe episodes of anxiety or depression as a normal adjustment reaction to change (very similar to a process of grief). "Adjusting" really means problem-solving, to find new solutions and new ways of thinking. This takes mental energy ("worry work") and time (usually several weeks).

N.B. Reassurance is rarely reassuring. Having professional carers who try to understand how you feel is reassuring.

Relaxation and massage can be a very effective iin managing anxiety, and may be more useful than drug treatment. The physiotherapist or complementary therapists may be able to provide this. Some faith healers are similarly effective by inducing deep relaxation.

A Family Meeting will often reduce anxiety, especially if there are communication problems within the family. The important principle is to ask every family member present how this illness is affecting their life – the feelings then emerge without the need to ask directly "How do you feel?".

Listening to the family with the patient, so that they can witness each other's concerns, can reduce the feeling of isolation for the patient, often brought about by feelings of mutual protectiveness within the family ("We didn't want to upset him").

A psychologist may be able to offer a series of appointments to help the person cope and to increase their understanding of how their thoughts affect their feelings ("cognitive therapy"). Some patients find it helpful to keep a diary of daily events, to understand what activities or thoughts trigger their morbid thoughts (see Psychological therapy).

Denial can be appropriate and helpful, especially if the patient has faced up to the situation, sorted out any affairs, and now prefers to forget about the disease ("non-attention" denial). Denial that is a used as a defense ("defensive denial") is due to fear, and may be an important defense mechanism at certain stages of adjustment, but the fear can escalate if it goes unchallenged, and the patient never benefits from facing and overcoming fears. Unrequested information must never be thrust upon the patient, but asking questions is helpful because it allows the patient to listen to his or her own words and this helps in the process of adjustment. Many professional carers make the incorrect assumption that asking questions about fears will worsen the fears, and important conversations are therefore avoided. It is always safe to ask questions in a relationship of trust (which can be established quickly, in some cases). Open-ended questions (What? Why? or How?) open up communication of feelings. The following questions can be helpful when exploring denial:

- How do you feel things are going at the moment?
- What have your other doctors told you ?
- How did you feel when the doctor told you it was an ulcer?
- What does your family know about your illness?

Allow time for the patient to ask questions. This enables you to judge the correct level of information that will help to reduce anxiety. Avoid giving information until you are certain that it is being requested. If you feel unsure how to respond, ask questions:

- Is that what you think\feel?
- Have you asked anyone else that question?
- I wonder why you are asking that question?

Further reading:
Stedeford A, Facing Death: Patients, Families and Professionals. London, Heinemann Medical Books, 1984

ASCITES

Ascites means fluid in the peritoneal cavity. It occurs in 6% of cancer patients. It is caused by malignant peritoneal deposits, blockage of sub-diaphragmatic lymphatics and secondary sodium retention. It occurs in cancers of the bronchus and breast, as well as intra-abdominal tumours, most commonly: ovary, colon, stomach, pancreas, bronchus, endometrium and cervix.

Symptoms of ascites includes:

- Abdominal discomfort
- Difficulty bending
- Heartburn
- Leg oedema
- Dyspnoea.

Diagnosis of ascites is based on:

- Abdominal distension
- Shifting dullness (detects 500ml)
- Ultrasound scan (detects 100ml)

Prognosis with ascites is about 40 days on average, but varies from 1-9 months. It can be relatively long with cancers of the breast and ovary. Ascites due to an unknown primary tumour usually has a poor prognosis but CT scan or even laparotomy may be indicated to exclude ovarian cancer which has a 70% response rate to chemotherapy.

Treatment options for ascites include:

- Analgesia
- Paracentesis
- Diuretics
- P-V shunt
- Intra-peritoneal chemotherapy
- Systemic chemotherapy (ovarian cancer)

Analgesia may be all that is required to overcome any discomfort or mild dsypnoea, although active patients usually want the fluid drained.

Paracentesis is a simple drainage procedure to reduce discomfort or dyspnoea. For an ambulant patient, the fluid can be removed rapidly in the outpatient clinic, 5-10 litres over 1-2 hours. In weaker patients it should be drained more slowly, as hypotension can occur. The fluid tends to re-accumulate over a period of 1-3 weeks, unless diuretics are used.

Diuretics will reduce malignant ascites over 2-3 weeks, provided high enough doses are used. Start with spironolactone 200mg plus frusemide 40mg daily, and if the patient tolerates these doses, double the dose after 1 week. Diuretics are effective because there is an element of sodium retention contributing to the ascites. A common management regime, suitable for outpatients, is to remove most of the fluid by paracentesis and to start the patient on high doses of diuretics to slow down the re-accumulation of the fluid. Monitor treatment of ascites by weekly abdominal girth measurement, and reduce the dose of diuretics once the ascites resolves, otherwise there is a risk of dehydration on such high doses.

In one study 13 out of 15 patients with malignant ascites achieved an excellent response to spironolactone, in a final dose of 150-450mg per day, with the ascites taking 10 days to 4 weeks to resolve, and 8 patients remained free of ascites for 1-4 months (Greenway, 1982). The patients had increased urinary sodium excretion levels, and the mechanism is assumed to be reversal of sodium retention (which may be due to ascites causing reduced circulating blood volume and increased renin levels).

IV Frusemide infusion (100mg over 24 hours by infusion pump at 5ml per hour) may be an alternative to paracentesis for the rapid relief of tense ascites. In one study 4 patients had a rapid and significant reduction in abdominal girth, partly due to a diuresis (1-3L over 24 hours) and possibly also due to re-distribution of fluid (Short report, BMJ 7 April 1984 Vol 288: p1041)

A peritoneo-venous shunt (P-V shunt) is indicated for a relatively fit patient troubled by recurrent ascites. This situation arises most commonly in patients with cancer of the breast or ovary. A shunt can provide excellent control of ascites, and should be considered at an early stage. A Denver shunt is commonly used, which has a valve and a reservoir which can be pumped. The shunt is easily inserted under a short general anaesthetic. The abdominal end is inserted into the hypochondrium and the venous end is led subcutaneously to a neck incision and inserted into the internal jugular vein. It is not indicated if the fluid is blood-stained or turbid, (because the shunt will quickly block) or if the fluid is loculated. Unfortunately 30% occlude within 3-6 months and need to be replaced.

Post mortem studies of 14 patients with shunts show that despite the infusion of viable malignant cells into the venous circulation, there is no development of clinically significant metastases. Such post-mortem studies may provide clues into the local factors that allow some organs to develop metastases and not others. For example in 7 patients with cancer of the ovary of the same histology, 2 had small, clinically insignificant, metastases, yet 5 had no metastases. (Reference: Tarin D et al. BMJ 10 March 1984, Vol 288, p 749-751)

The procedure of paracentesis involves:

- Diagnose fluid (consider ultrasound)
- Empty bladder
- Use 0.5% bupivacaine (Marcain)
- Keep 10cm from the midline (to avoid blood vessels)
- Insert cannula in left or right iliac fossa.

A paediatric thoracic trocar and cannula (Portex 10FG) is recommended for paracentesis, as it has several advantages. It is fenestrated, so it rarely blocks; it fits tightly onto the tube of an ordinary urinary catheter bag (preventing leaks) and it is a narrow gauge, so a purse-string suture is not usually needed. It has a slightly bulbous tip, and a sharp-tipped scalpel has to be used to make a track through to the peritoneum, once the skin is anaesthetized. If fluid does dribble out of the puncture site, a colostomy bag can be used to collect the fluid, which usually stops draining within a few hours. (Warn the patient that this may occur and reassure that it is harmless).

Intra-peritoneal chemotherapy is logical in that a significantly higher drug concentration is achieved than following IV administration, and because patients with malignant ascites have a reduced peritoneal clearance rate for drugs. In one study 7 out of 16 patients had a complete response, with no re-accumulation of ascites for 60 days, after 90mg bleomycin was given in a large volume of fluid (2 litres saline) – after the ascites had been drained to dryness. The patient was tipped head down and turned side to side and the fluid was then drained off after 15-30 minutes to reduce the risk of adhesions. The main side-effect is fever which can be reduced by giving IV hydrocortisone 100mg at the same time.

Other cytotoxics can be instilled, and a variety of agents have been used, including 5-flurouracil, thiotepa, and quinacrine but in practice they are disappointing and rarely indicated. Studies mostly show a "partial response" rate of around 30% for these agents.

Targeted antibody therapy (Radio-immuno-therapy) is a novel approach to the management of ascites, that has achieved useful palliation in some cases. Monoclonal antibodies to tumour antigens (detected on malignant cells in the fluid) are coupled to a radio-isotope (I-131) and given intraperitoneally to deliver radiation directly to tumour-bearing areas.

References:
Greenway B, Johnson PJ, Williams R, Control of Malignant Ascites with spironolactone. Br J Surg 1982; 69: 441-442.
Ostrowski MJ, Assessment of the lonterm results of controlling the reaccumulation of malignant effusions using intracavity bleomycin, Cancer 1986; 57: 721-7).

BLADDER CANCER

Bladder cancer causes around 5,500 deaths per year in the UK. It is associated with smoking and has been linked to certain industrial chemicals (benzidine, napthylamine) used in the chemical, rubber and cable industries. Peak age is 50-70 and it is twice as common in men.

Presentation is typically with painless haematuria (sometimes with dysuria or suprapubic ache). Cystoscopy and CT scan are performed to diagnose and stage the disease.

Early disease (stage 1) confined to the mucosa, is treated with diathermy, laser or instillations of chemotherapeutic drugs, but 50% eventually recur, therefore follow-up cystoscopies are needed. If the tumour has invaded muscle wall (stage 2 and 3) only 30% survive 5 years. Treatment is then by one of the following:

- Partial cystectomy (if the tumour is small and a bladder capacity of 300ml can be left)
- Radical radiotherapy (60 Gy over 6 weeks)
- Total cystectomy with an ileal conduit (a pouch of ileum, with blood supply, brought out as a stoma, with the ureters implanted into it)

Advanced disease (stage 4) involving pelvic or para-aortic nodes, or fixation to vagina or rectum has a poor prognosis of a few months. Palliative radiotherapy (e.g. 35 Gy over 10 days) may be given to control haematuria (effective in 50%), but may cause urinary frequency.
Metastases occur to bone (most commonly) peritoneum (causing ascites), lung and liver.

Chemotherapy is considered for recurrent disease after surgery or radiotherapy that is causing severe symptoms of pain or lymphoedema, but not for asymptomatic metastases (such as in the lung). Combinations of methotrexate, vinblastine, doxorubicin and cisplatin give high response rates around 45% for a median of 20 weeks, but side-effects can be severe. Treatment is monitored by CT scan and if there is no response after 2 cycles it should be stopped.

Problems in advanced cancer of the bladder include.

- Visceral pain (suprapubic)
- Sciatic nerve pain (*see nerve pain*)
- Bladder spasms
- Frequency and dysuria
- Bladder haemorrhage
- Lymphoedema of the leg
- Ureteric obstruction

Bladder spasms are usually due to mucosal irritation at the trigone, causing attacks of severe suprapubic pain radiating into the urethra and perineum. Exclude infection. Treatment options include: oxybutinin 5mg TID, buscopan SC infusion 180mg\24 hours, bladder instillation of 0.5% bupivacaine 20ml for 20 minutes (*see Pain*).

Bladder haemorrhage may be controlled by radiotherapy, laser or hydrostatic dilatation, but for most hospice patients the best options are usually 1% alum bladder irrigation or oral tranexamic acid (*see Bleeding*).

Ureteric obstruction will cause rapidly cause renal failure and death if bilateral. It is suspected from a rising urea and creatinine. In a relatively fit patient it may be an indication for ureteric stent or a nephrostomy. Consider early referral to a urologist (*see Interventional radiology*).

BLEEDING

Troublesome bleeding occurs in about 15% of patients with advanced cancer. Treatment options include:

- Radiotherapy
- Laser therapy
- Embolization
- Cryotherapy
- Topical adrenaline
- Haemostatic dressings
- Tranexamic acid
- 1% alum
- Sucralfate
- Ethamsylate
- Platelet transfusion
- Vitamin K
- Russell Viper Venom

Radiotherapy may be the best way of controlling bleeding from advanced cutaneous tumours, especially fungating breast or ulcerated lymph nodes, provided there has been no previous RT to the area. Sensitive areas such as perineum or vulva tolerate RT less well due to skin reactions. Radiotherapy will control haemoptysis in 90% of cases and is also effective for bleeding from the oesophagus, rectum, bladder, kidney, vagina and uterus. RT is usually given by external beam, but but intrauterine and intra-vaginal sources may be used, and intra-luminal radiotherapy can control bleeding from the oesophagus and bronchus, using a single 30 minute treatment as a day case.

Laser Therapy, via endoscopy, can control haemorrhage from lung, stomach, bladder and rectal cancers (*see Lasers*).

Embolization of bleeding arteries may be possible at a wide variety of sites, by means of transcatheter angiography under local anaesthetic and the injection of gelatin or other inert substances. Useful sites for embolization include the internal iliac artery for bleeding from bladder or gynaecological tumours, and the renal artery for heavy renal bleeding. Embolization may be possible at other sites including stomach and lung, but the skills of interventional radiology are needed (*see Interventional radiology*).

1% Alum solution has to be freshly made up. for bladder haemorrhage it is given by continuous irrigation via a 3-way catheter, at a rate of 5ml per minute, ie 300ml per hour or 1L per 10 hours. With a small bladder capacity the patient may only tolerate smaller volumes, such as 1L per day, because of pain, but this can still be effective. Bleeding usually stops in 1-2 days. It works by precipitating protein on the mucosal surface and constricting capillaries. It is painless and does not require anaesthetic. It is non-toxic. It is more effective and easier to use than other agents, such as formalin or silver nitrate. 1% alum may be useful in other sites including rectal tumours or surface malignancies.

Preparation of 1% alum solution is by making a 60% solution in water, when it is necessary to heat the solution to make it dissolve, then take 50ml of the supersaturated solution and add to a 3 litre bag of sterile water for irrigation, filtering through a 0.22 micron filter in sterile conditions.

Platelet transfusions are rarely indicated because the effect is short-lived, but may have a place in a patient with marrow failure who has distressing bleeding, such as retinal or heavy nosebleeds.

Vitamin K (phytomenadione) 1–5mg by slow IV injection reverses warfarin within hours, by re-synthesis of clotting factors. Immediate reversal requires fresh frozen plasma. Warfarin should normally be stopped before the terminal phase of illness, because terminal gastric bleeding can sometimes occur, which can cause altered blood to trickle from the mouth as the patient dies, which is very distressing for relatives. However, it can be difficult chosing a right time to stop warfarin with patients on longterm anti-coagulation, who have been warned that it must never be stopped, such as those with heart valves, and since it takes several days for warfarin's anti-coagulation effect to wear off, vitamin K may be indicated.

Russell Viper Venom is very rarely needed (I have personally never used it) but is worth knowing about, in the event of heavy distressing surface bleeding. It is a very powerful clotting agent that converts prothrombin to thrombin. (It is an enzyme usually only used in the haematology laboratory, to investigate clotting disorders.)

Blood Transfusion tends to worsen active bleeding, and is only indicated if the bleeding is controlled.

Surface bleeding may be controlled by radiotherapy, adrenaline 1 in 1000, 1% alum, alginate dressings, tranexamic acid or sucralfate paste. Topical Adrenaline (1 in 1000), applied with light pressure, is a useful first-aid measure. Remove clots first. Alginate dressings (Kaltostat, Sorbsan) are haemostatic for surface bleeding. Tranexamic acid (Cyclocapron) tablets or syrup, 500mg, Q.I.D. will effectively control capilliary bleeding. Sucralfate (Antepsin) made into a paste with KY jelly can also be effective. Sucralfate contains aluminium.

Haematuria: Treatment options include:

- Total cystectomy
- Radiotherapy to bladder or kidney
- 1% Alum bladder washouts
- Clot removal
- Hydrostatic balloon distension
- Cystoscopic laser.
- Renal embolization
- Oral Tranexamic acid
- Oral ethamsylate

Light haematuria needs no action, other than explanation. Exclude infection. Citrate bladder washouts can dissolve small clots. Consider oral iron therapy. Red discolouration can be caused by danthron (co-danthramer, co-danthrusate). Dark discolouration may be due to bile or dehydration.

Heavy bleeding is best controlled by irrigating the bladder with 1% Alum Solution, in a patient unfit for surgery. Radiotherapy to control renal haemorrhage can be considered providing the contralateral kidney is functioning. Radiotherapy for bladder haemorrhage is only possible if the patient has not already received RT to contol the cancer. Cystoscopic removal of large clots can sometimes control bleeding. Hydrostatic distension for 10-20 minutes under GA applies local pressure and can be effective. Diathermy tends to worsen bleeding. Laser therapy is effective but only-available in special centres. Embolization of the renal artery can control renal haemorrhage but severe pain and fever can occur after the proceedure. Oral tranexamic acid can be effective for light bleeding but there is a risk of causing clot formation. Encourage a high fluid intake, and start with a low dose (500mg BD) and increase slowly depending on effect. Oral ethamsylate (Dicynene) 500mg QID enhances platelet adhesiveness and is excreted unchanged in urine, and may reduce light bleeding.

Visceral (internal) bleeding may be controlled by radiotherapy or laser therapy. Oral tranexamic acid can control light visceral bleeding. It should be used cautiously for bladder haemorrhage, as is a danger of hard clots forming in the bladder that need to be removed cystoscopically. It may take several days for the bleeding to stop completely. Rectal bleeding from a carcinoma may be controlled with a tranexamic acid enema, 5g in 50ml warm water, twice a day (Lancet 1991; 337, 431). Alternatively 1% Alum solution can be used as an enema (Br J Surg. 1986; 73: 192). N.B. Upper G.I. bleeds are more commonly due to gastritis, peptic ulceration or haemorrhagic oesophagitis than due to malignancy.

Nosebleeds are usually venous. Bleeds from anterior to the nasal septum (Little's area) can often be stopped by direct pressure, by pinching the nostrils for 10 minutes. If bleeding continues into the nasopharynx then the site is more posterior, and may require balloon catheter or packing with BIPP gauze (Bismuth iodoform paraffin paste). Recurrent small bleeds may require cauterization under local anaesthetic. Consider checking the Hb after heavy bleeds are controlled. Treatment can be summarized as:

- External pressure (15minutes)
- Pack with ribbon gauze soaked in 1% Alum
- Refer to ENT department for:
- 3-day bismuth-iodine pack, or
- Diathermy under direct inspection
- ?Platelet transfusion (leukaemia)

Heavy Arterial Bleeding may occur from erosion of the aorta (massive haemoptysis) or carotid artery (head and neck cancers) or axillary or femoral arteries (malignant nodes). It may be a terminal event. Management involves:

- ?Resuscitate (IV line, X-match)
- Someone to stay <u>with</u> patient
- Sedation if agitated, with:
  - IV or IM diamorphine, or
  - IV Diazemuls 5-10mg,or
  - IM midazolam 1mg into deltoid
- Green surgical towels (reduces visual impact)
- Support for observers (including other patients)

References:
Regnard C, Makin W. Management of bleeding in advanced cancer – a flow diagram. Palliative Medicine 1992; 6: 65-73
Reidy JF. Stopping bleeding by embolization, Br Med J 1987; 294: 592 3.

BONE PAIN

Bone pain is due to metastatic destruction of bone. It causes 40% of cancer pain. 80% of cases are due to cancers of the breast, <u>bronchus or prostate</u>. The incidence of bone metastases in these tumours is:

- Bronchus 30%
- Breast 70%
- Prostate 85%

Cancers of the kidney, thyroid, pancreas, stomach, colon, ovary, melanoma and myeloma also spread to bone. 75% of myeloma patients present with bone pain.

The mechanism of bone pain remains poorly understood. Pain is thought to be due to release of prostaglandins (especially E1 and E2) which sensitize the nerve endings to pain-producing chemicals. Nerve fibres are present in the periosteum, but not the cortex or medullary cavity. Pain does not correlate with the number or size of bone metastases. The mechanism of pain relief following RT, hypophysectomy or calcitonin is probably chemical, since it occurs too quickly for tumour shrinkage to have occured.

<u>Bone is not destroyed by cancer cells</u>. Tumour peptides increase osteoclastic activity and bone destruction with a secondary increase in bone formation by osteoblasts (causing a rise in alkaline phosphatase levels). Tumour peptides disturb the normal balance of bone remodelling, with excessive osteoclastic cavity formation (osteolytic metastases) or excessive osteoblastic activity (sclerotic metastases). Osteoblasts lay down osteoid in a haphazard way that does not strengthen the bone structure. Biphosphonates inhibit osteoclastic bone resorbtion and may come to have

a place in the management of some bone metastases, by slowing down bone destruction.

The commonest sites of bone metastases are:

- Spine (lumbar and thoracic)
- Pelvis
- Ribs

Other sites of bone metastases are skull, cervical spine, femur and humerus (especially in cancer of the kidney).

Bone marrow infiltration is rare in solid tumours, which mainly affect cortical bone. About 1% of Breast cancer involves bone marrow. Marrow replacement results in anaemia, bleeding (low platelet count) and infection (low white cell count) In solid tumours marrow involvement usually means the prognosis is very poor.

Clinical features of bone pain are:

- Pain on movement ("incident pain")
- Relieved by rest
- Well-localized pain
- Continuous ache (if severe)
- Bony tenderness on pressure
- Pathological fractures

Bone pain is typically worse on movement, well-localized and tender to pressure or percussion. Occasionally the pain can be poorly localized and with no obvious bony tenderness. Vertebral compression may occur and cause radiating nerve root pains around both sides of the chest.

Diagnosis of bone metastases can be confirmed by:

- Xrays
- Bone scan
- CT scan
- MRI scan
- Biopsy (if diagnosis is uncertain)

Metastases are usually multiple. A solitary lesion is more likely to be benign and bone biopsy may be then be indicated. Xrays detect metastases of 4mm diameter, when there is at least 50% trabecular bone erosion. Radionuclide bone scans are more sensitive but less specific than X-rays. They show any areas of oseoblastic activity as "hot spots", which may be due to metastases or arthritis, (but the difference is usually clinically obvious). Lesions as small as 1–2cm can be detected. The lytic lesions of myeloma or renal cancer do not show on an isotope bone scan, but will show on a CT scan. An MRI scan will also show any associated soft-tissue involvement or marrow infiltration.

Treatment options for bone pain include:

- Radiotherapy
- Hemi-body irradiation
- Radioactive Strontium
- NSAIDs
- Morphine (for continuous ache)
- Internal fixation
- Chemotherapy\Hormones
- Calcitonin
- Biphosphonates

Radiotherapy is the treatment of choice for bone pain. 80% of patients get a response (50% complete, 30% partial) sometimes within 1-2 days, and 30% within 1 week, but occasionally pain relief takes 3-4 weeks to occur. Radiotherapy can control bone pain irrespective of the histology of the metastasis, even if the primary tumour is radio-resistant (e.g. melanoma).

A single treatment (8 Gy) can give as good pain relief as multiple fractions, regardless of histology, and is preferred for some sites (eg long bones) in patients with a short prognosis. In one prospective study of 288 patients with bone pain, randomized to receive either 8 Gy in a single treatment or 30 Gy in 10 daily fractions, there was no difference in speed of onset of pain relief or duration of onset, and independent of the histology of the primary tumour. There was no difference in ealry or late morbidity. For patients with a short prognosis it is advantageous to use few fractions whenever possible (Price et al, 1986).

Multiple fractions are preferred if there is any risk of damage to the spinal cord or nerve roots, and will cause less nausea, vomiting and diarrhoea when the field includes the bowel. In patients with a longer prognosis a fractionated course may be preferred because the tumour killing effect is greater and may reduce the need for later retreatment.

Hemibody irradiation can be used if painful metastases are scattered over widespread parts of the body. (This is occasionally seen in carcinoma of the prostate and in myeloma). 8 Gy are given as a single dose over a wide field, to either the upper or lower half of the body. 80% get pain relief within 1-2 days. The patient needs to be admitted, and pre-medicated with steroids and anti-emetics, because malaise, vomiting and neutropenia can all be severe, and the white cell count must be carefully monitored for the next 10 days, and haematological support may be needed. The proceedure can be repeated to the opposite half of the body after an interval of 6 weeks. Local areas of bone pain that occur at later can still be treated with radiotherapy.

Bone-seeking isotopes such as intravenous radio-active Strontium (87Sr) concentrate in areas of high osteoblastic activity. They can be used to treat multiple painful bone metastases. It delivers a relatively low dose to a widespread area and about 70% get a response within 1-2 days. It can be repeated. Local sites can still be treated with external palliative radiotherapy.

NSAIDs (Non-Steroidal Anti-Inflammatory Drugs) are prostaglandin inhibitors and will control bone pain in 80% of cases within a few days. They block prostaglandin synthesis by inhibiting the enzyme cyclo-oxygenase. There are no comparative trials demonstrating the relative efficacy of NSAIDs. Naproxen (Naprosyn) 500mg BD is often the first choice, and is available as tablets, suspension or suppositories. Unfortunately all NSAIDs have a 20% incidence of gastric irritation. This can be reduced by giving ranitidine 150mg BD simultaneously, (or misoprostol or omeprazole – *see Dyspepsia*). Patients who develop side-effects with one NSAID may be able to tolerate another. (*see NSAIDs*). The response to NSAIDs is:

- 60% to any NSAID
- 20% on changing the NSAID
- 20% do not respond

Morphine is not helpful for bone pain on movement, and is only helpful if there is a continuous aching element to the pain. The sharp pains on movement ("incident pain") are not relieved by morphine.

Internal fixation may be required for large metastases of the femur, especially if there is a lot of cortical bone damage, to reduce pain and to reduce the risk of fracture. Some special centres perform more aggressive prosthetic surgery for bone metastases (*see Fractures*).

Chemotherapy\Hormone therapy can control bone pain, but may take several weeks to be effective, and other methods of pain control (RT or NSAIDs) will usually be needed as well. Hormone therapy controls pain in cancer of the prostate (60-90% response rate) or breast (20-50%). Chemotherapy may be effective in small cell lung cancer, breast cancer or myeloma. The response rates and duration of pain relief tend to be lower with chemotherapy than hormone therapy.

Calcitonin inhibits osteoclastic bone resorbtion, and is normally used to treat hypercalcaemia and bone pain in Paget's disease, but has also been used to treat malignant bone pain. Salcalcitonin (Calsynar), 400 i.u. is given twice a day for 2 days (4 doses). It is advisable to give anti-emetics simultaneously, because calcitonin can cause severe nausea and vomiting. There is no need to monitor calcium levels.

Biphosphonates may come to have a place in the treatment of bone pain. They are enzyme-resistant analogues of pyrophosphate which inhibit osteoclastic activity. They are mainly used to treat hypercalcaemia, but may come to have a clinical place in treating bone pain that does not respond to radiotherapy or NSAIDs, or slowing the progession of lytic metastases. They are poorly absorbed orally. In one study, fortnightly infusions of 30mg of pamidronate were given to patients with breast cancer with bone metastases and found to reduce bone pain; there was some evidence that it also slowed the progression of the bone metastases. It is not necessary to monitor calcium levels.

References:
Price P *et al*. Prospective randomized trial of single and multifraction radiotherapy schedules in the treatment of painful bony metastases, Radiotherapy and Oncology 1986, 6: 247-255
Bates TD. The management of bone metastases: radiotherapy Palliative Medicine 1987; 1: 117-120.
Dodwell D, Howell A, Treating bone metastases. Br Med J 1991; 303: 429-30.

BRAIN METASTASES

Brain metastases occur in about 10% of cancer patients. The median survival with brain metastases is about 4 months. Brain metastases are multiple in at least 80% of cases. The sites of spread are most commonly the cerebral hemispheres (80%) but occasionally other parts of the brain are involved: cerebellum (15%), Pituitary (6%) and brain stem (1%).

Tumours that cause brain metastases are most commonly cancers of the bronchus and breast, but many other tumours occasionally spread to brain, including melanoma, renal, gastro-intestinal, genito-urinary and others.

Clinical features of brain metastases include:

- Headaches, vomiting (raised ICP)
- Weakness, inco-ordination
- Speech difficulties
- Hemianopia (loss of peripheral vision)
- Incontinence
- Intellectual damage
- Siezures (25%)

Brain metastases can initially mimic a stroke, with sudden onset of weakness or dysphasia, but the signs tend to gradually worsen ("step-wise progression") whereas a stroke gradually improves.

High dose steroids (dexamethasone 16mg daily) improve the symptoms in 75% of patients, usually for 1-2 months. They reduce the peri-tumour oedema, but do not affect the cancer cells, and the effect wears off. Steroids are of most benefit for metastatic tumours and high grade astrocytomas, but less use for slow-growing, infiltrating tumours. It is reasonable to start with 16mg dexamethasone daily. A loading dose is unnecessary, as a steady plasma level is achieved within 24 hours.

Clinical improvement on steroids, if it is to occur, is usually seen within 24 hours, but it may be reasonable to try higher doses (32mg daily) for 2-3 days. If a response occurs, the patient is then maintained on a dose that has to be individually determined. Reduction below the correct maintainance dose causes neurological deterioration. The dose is reduced slowly by about 2mg per week, in order to reduce the risk of side-effects, but if the symptoms recur, the dose should be increased again. A second response to steroids is unusual, and deterioration on steroids is usually taken as a signal to consider stopping them. It is best to decide in advance of starting steroids what the desired response is, and to stop steroids again if it is not achieved.

Continuing steroids, as the patient's condition starts deteriorating, may seem inappropriate, in case the steroids are prolonging dying. On the other hand, the family may fear that reducing the dose may actively shorten life. In fact both fears are usually unjustified, and the end stage of the disease takes much the same course, with or without steroids. One solution is to continue steroids until the patient is no longer able to swallow them.

What is the correct dose of steroids? An outline history of steroid dosage for brain tumours shows that the routine starting dose of 16mg daily is arbitrary, and a higher dose may be indicated at times. In 1957 a patient with brain metastases was noted to have a rapid neurological improvement with prednisolone (given as endocrine therapy for breast cancer). In 1961 dexamthasone was used to reduce cerebral oedema, when the dose chosen was an arbitrary 10mg IV and then 4mg 6 hourly. In 1973, in a study of patients on 16mg of dexamethasone daily, (following partial excision of brain tumours) 11 out of 20 patients who were deterioratating on 16 mg had useful improvement by increasing the dose of dexamethasone as high as 96mg daily (but 4 did not respond even at that dose).

The mechanism of action of steroids remains poorly understood. CT scan shows a halo of oedema around a tumour, due to leakage of protein-rich exudate from capillaries. This increases brain volume, which can be only partly compensated for by a reduction in CSF and blood volume. Dexamethasone causes cerebral vasoconstriction and reduces cerebral blood volume, which probably accounts for its action. Vasodilators such as nitrates should be avoided as they may increase the pressure by cerebral vasodilatation (see Steroids).

Cranial irradiation of the whole brain is considered for relatively fit patients who develop brain metastases with no evidence of metastases elsewhere. This situation occurs most commonly with carcinoma of the breast. RT increases the median survival from around 4 weeks to 4-6 months. 50% of patients get neurological improvement for a median of 3 months. Hair loss occurs (and the hair re-grows) but there are no other side-effects. A randomized multi-centre trial is currently comparing 12Gy in 2 fractions with 30Gy in 10 fractions.

Neurosurgery is only considered if there is a solitary metastasis in a relatively fit patient with no evidence of metastases elsewhere. 50% survive 1 year, 20% survive 2 years.

Further reading:
Kirkham SR, The palliation of cerebral tumours with high dose dexamethasone: a review, Palliative Medicine 1988; 2: 27-33

BREAST CANCER

Breast cancer is the most prevalent cancer in the UK, affecting 1 in 12 women. It causes 15,000 deaths per year in the UK. The risk is 3X higher with a family history in first degree relatives. Breast cancer is increasingly seen as a systemic disease from the outset, the control of micrometastases being the key to longterm survival.

Presentation of breast cancer is usually as a painless lump (less commonly nipple discharge or inversion). Diagnosis is by biopsy (needle or excision). Most are poorly differentiated adenocarcinomas, arising from the ducts.

Treatment of breast cancer by simple mastectomy or "lumpectomy" followed by RT is as effective as extended surgery for small tumours (less than 4cm) in terms of both local control and survival. There is growing evidence that adjuvant therapy (to treat the micrometastases assumed to be present) with tamoxifen or chemotherapy can reduce the risk of recurrence.

Prognosis is better if the there is a long disease-free interval, if the patient is over 60, and with oestrogen receptor positive tumours. Once axillary nodes are involved ("node positive, scan negative" disease) 60% will develop metastases, usually within 5 years (but occasionally 10-20 years later).

Metastases most commonly occur to bone, but also to distant nodes, brain, lung, pleura, liver, peritoneum, and skin. Metastases are often confined to bone in older patients. Metastatic disease has a median survival of 3 years with good palliative treatment, and 10% survive 5 years.

Hormone therapy will produce a response in 45% of patients. Bone, lung and nodal disease tend to respond better than liver or brain. No clear guidelines are yet available for the optimum use of hormones in breast cancer (*see Hormone therapy*).

Chemotherapy in breast cancer may be indicated for failure of hormone therapy (or oophorectomy), aggressive visceral disease (lungs or liver) or local disease not amenable to RT or surgery. As with hormone therapy, bone, lung and nodal disease tend to respond better than liver or brain. If both treatments are given together it improves initial response rate slightly but not survival. A commonly used combination is cyclophosphamide, methotrexate and fluorouracil (CMF). Other drugs that have an established place include doxorubicin (hair loss), mitomycin (marrow suppression) and mitozantrone. There are no clear data supporting the use of combinations over single agents. 50% respond for a median of 6 months (sometimes for 9-12 months) and Xrays may be helpful to monitor response. The optimum duration of chemotherapy is not known. If a response occurs treatment is usually continued for 6 months and then stopped (longterm treatment does not improve survival). If a second course of treatment is given the response rate falls to around 20% for 2-3 months. If the disease progresses during chemotherapy then it is stopped.

One study has shown that chemotherapy does improve well being, mood, pain control, appetite and overall quality of life in advanced breast cancer, and that 6 months treatment gives better results than 3 months (Coates A et al, N Eng J Med 1987; 317: 1490-5).

Problems in advanced cancer of the breast may include:

- Arm lymphoedema – 30%
- Pleural effusion
- Ascites
- Brain metastases -20%
- Chest wall recurrence – 10%
- Cranial nerve palsies – 10%
- Hypercalcaemia – 5%

Locally advanced disease should be controlled if possible, to improve quality of life, and can be treated with radiotherapy, surgery or tamoxifen. 15% will survive 5 years. Good control of the disease can be obtained in 3-4 weeks after radiotherapy. Mastectomy ("toilet mastectomy") may still offer good palliation for certain patients, even if metastases are already present.

Cranial nerve palsies are typical of advanced breast disease, and commonly cause double vision, facial numbness or weakness of the tongue. They can respond well to radiotherapy to the base of the skull.

Brain metastases are usually multiple. They tend to respond poorly to hormone therapy or chemotherapy. Whole brain irradiation should be considered for relatively fit patients with troublesome neurological problems. It is not considered if the patient's condition is deteriorating rapidly. Patients who show a good response to steroids will respond to cranial irradiation, when 75% improve for 3-6 months, and median survival is doubled to 4 months, with 10% of patients surviving a year. The whole brain is irradiated because of the high probability of multiple metastases. Hair loss occurs, (but re-grows over several weeks) and there are few other side-effects if steroids are given simultaneously. A relatively high dose can be used (3000cGy over 10 days) because brain cells do not divide, although if the patient should survive 2 years a dementia-like syndrome can occur.

BUBBLING

Terminal bubbling (death rattle) is usually more distressing for the relatives than the patient. It is not always possible to control the bubbling noise with drugs.

Turning or re-positioning the patient sometimes stops the bubbling for a time.

Atropine can be used if the patient is still conscious and does not want to be made any more drowsy. 0.6mg every 4-6 hours orally or IM or by subcutaneous infusion.

Hyoscine (scopolamine) hydrobromide 0.4mg 4 hourly IM or 1.6-2.4mg by SC infusion over 24 hours will dry secretions. Hyoscine is also very sedating, which can be an advantage if the patient is restless.

Glycopyronium bromide (Robinul) is a powerful anticholinergic, and an alternative to hyoscine. 0.2mg 6 hourly or 0.8mg by SC infusion over 24 hours may control bubbling if hyoscine is ineffective.

Scopaderm patches each contain a low dose of hyoscine hydrobromide, 0.5mg, released over 3 days. It takes 6 hours to reach peak plasma levels. The adhesive plaster is stuck to an area of hairless skin, usually behind the ear. It is intended for motion sickness, and 2-3 patches are usually needed simultaneously to have any effect on respiratory secretions.

Frusemide 40-80mg IM will sometimes reduce bubbling when the anti-cholinergic drugs are not effective. The patient should be catheterized because the combination of a diuretic and anti-cholinergic drugs is likely to cause retention.

The family are often distressed by the noise, and always appreciate explanation. The following points about the bubbling noise can be made and are often reassuring:

- Fluid in the airways
- Unable to cough due to weakness
- Patient not aware of bubbling
- More distressing for the watching relatives

CANCER STATISTICS

Cancer is responsible for a quarter of all deaths, 160,000 deaths per year in the UK.

Cancer deaths per year in the UK (1989) – figures from Cancer Research Campaign.

Lung	40,223
Breast	15,381
Large bowel	12,969
Stomach	10,612
Unknown primary	10,000
Prostate	8,234
Pancreas	6,796
Rectum	6,483

Oesophagus	5,591
Bladder	5,358
Ovary	4,274
Leukaemia	4,084
Lymphoma	3,063
Brain	2,940
Kidney	2,667
Myeloma	2,373
Cervix	2,170
Hepatoma	1,607
Uterus (body)	1,030
Melanoma	1,192
Larynx	953
Sarcoma	600
Vulva	500
Mouth	489
Hodgkin's	483
Thyroid	398
Small gut	280
Testis	152
All other types	14,000

The 10 commonest cancers in men are: lung, prostate, stomach, colon, bladder, rectum, oesophagus, pancreas, leukaemia and brain.

The 10 commonest cancers in women are: breast, lung, colon, stomach, ovary, pancreas, rectum, oesophagus, cervix and leukaemia.

Smoking is thought to cause about 30% of all cancers including most lung cancer and a proportion of deaths from cancers of mouth, pharynx, larynx, oesophagus, bladder, cervix leukaemia, probably pancreas and possibly kidney.

Survival for most cancers in the UK has changed little in the past 20 years. Average 5 year survival figures for cancers at all stages of development (for 1981) are:

Uterus	70%
Breast	62%
Bladder	62%
Cervix	58%
Prostate	46%
Colon	37%
Rectum	36%
Ovary	28%
Leukaemia	29%
Stomach	10%
Bronchus	7%
Oesophagus	7%
Pancreas	4%

Survival depends on many factors (stage, histology and possibly psychological), therefore these figures are less meaningful for individuals. Treatment at an early stage improves survival, e.g. early treatment of breast cancer has a survival of over 80%. Some less common cancers have a 5 year survival rate over 50%, including sarcomas, eye tumours, Hodgkin's disease, melanoma and cancers of the larynx, placenta, testis and thyroid.

50% of cancers are not curable even at the time of diagnosis, when treatment (surgery, radiotherapy, and chemotherapy) aims to palliate (control symptoms and prolong life) rather than cure. In advanced disease the aim becomes control of symptoms and enhancement of the quality of remaining life (hospice style care). Metastatic disease causes many similar symptoms and problems regardless of the primary site of the tumour. However, individual cancers may cause additional specific problems, outlined in separate sections throughout the book.

CERVICAL CANCER

Cancer of the cervix causes around 2000 deaths per year in the UK. It is preventable by screening with regular cervical smears, provided abnormal smears are followed up by colposcopy, and areas of dysplasia are treated (by laser or cryotherapy). If dysplasia is left untreated for several years, 30-40% will progress to invasive cancer.

Presentation is typically with abnormal vaginal bleeding (post-coital or post-menopausal). Pain or urinary symptoms suggest advanced disease. Patients presenting with advanced disease (stage 4) can be treated with palliative radiotherapy or chemotherapy (methotrexate or cisplatinum), to reduce symptoms such as pain or discharge, but any response is usually short-lived.

95% of cervical cancer is squamous (5% are adenocarcinomas, which tend to spread into the uterus and are best treated surgically). For disease confined to the cervix (stage 1) a Wertheim's hysterectomy or radiotherapy will cure 90%.

Radiotherapy can still cure 50% when pelvic nodes are involved (stage 2) and 30% where spread has reached the pelvic side-walls (stage 3). is given both internally by Caesium insertion (to treat the cervix) and by external beam irradiation (to treat pelvic nodes). Radiotherapy causes ablation of the ovaries and a premature menopause, so HRT is be needed if the patient is pre-menopausal. Vaginal stenosis occurs with RT, and patients are advised to practise regular intercourse or use vaginal dilators during and after treatment.

Recurrent cancer of the cervix is suspected if there is pain, leg swelling (lymphoedema) or urinary symptoms and is confirmed by CT scan which may also show hydronephrosis. Recurrence after surgery can be treated, and occasionally cured, by radiotherapy (*see Pelvic Recurrence*).

Chemotherapy is used to treat symptoms such as pain or lymphoedema due to progress of the disease. It is a relatively chemo-sensitive tumour, and combinations of bleomycin, ifosfamide, cisplatin and methotrexate can achieve responses of around 60% for a median of 5-6 months. Side-effects can be severe, and chemotherapy is not justified if there are no symptoms, since the effect on survival is not signigicant. Response is assessed by CT scan, ultrasound scan and examination under anaesthetic. If there is no response in symptoms after 2 cycles it should be abandoned.

Problems in advanced cancer of the cervix include:

- Pain
- Discharge, bleeding
- Fistulas
- Leg lymphoedema
- Ureteric obstruction
- Hypercalcaemia (5%)
- Psychological issues

Pain from pelvic tumours can be of various types (*see Pelvic recurrence*).

Radiotherapy or chemotherapy may be used to shrink the tumour, and control symtoms, especially for patients who presented with advanced disease and have not yet had cancer treatment.

Discharge may be profuse and foul smelling. Metronidazole can reduce smell, tranexamic acid can control any bleeding. Change dressings regularly. Continuous dribbling suggests a vesico-vaginal fistula, and leak of faecal material suggests a recto-vaginal fistula. Palliative surgery (ileal diversion or colostomy) should be considered whenever possible for these distressing symptoms. Explanation and support can reduce guilt and isolation.

Psychological issues (especially guilt and anger) may be due to the association with sexual intercourse (possibly linked to a human papillomavirus) or to the fact that the disease may have been preventable with effective screening.

Recurrence or RT damage? Radiotherapy can cause small bowel damage, (with stenosis and obstruction) or fistulas (from the rectum or bladder into the vagina). The patient may require bowel resections, colostomy or urinary diversion, (and sometimes all three). When these complications arise, recurrent cancer is often suspected, but as time passes and the patient's condition remains stable, the true diagnosis becomes apparent. CT scan is often unhelpful, because it is difficult to distinguish areas of radiation fibrosis from recurrent cancer.

Reference:
Williams C. Current issues in cancer. Br Med J 1992; 304: 1501-4.

CHEMOTHERAPY

Curative chemotherapy is a possiblility for leukaemia, testicular cancer, Hodgkin's and high-grade lymphomas and some childhood cancers. Toxic effects are worthwhile if there is a chance of cure.

Palliative chemotherapy aims to control symptoms and improve quality of life. The evidence that it does so is difficult to find. The outcome of chemotherapy is usually measured in terms of tumour response. A response means regression of measurable lesions on skin or on Xrays. Palliative chemotherapy is used for the following tumours (response rates in brackets):

- Small cell lung cancer (75% respond)
- Breast (50%)
- Ovary (40%)
- Colo-rectal (20%)
- Stomach, (20%)
- Head and Neck (20%)
- Cervix (15%)
- Bladder (15%)
- Melanoma (5-10%)
- Sarcoma (5-10%)

"Will it make me feel better?" is the key question for many patients. Modern trials of palliative chemotherapy should assess the effect on the patient's symptoms and quality of life, which can sometimes be improved even when there is no evidence of measurable tumour response (Rakowsky *et al*, 1991).

Chemotherapy is not standard treatment for non-small cell lung cancers, or cancers of the prostate, oesophagus, liver, pancreas, vulva, endometrium, kidney and thyroid. Cytotoxic drugs should only be used in these tumours as part of a clinical trial.

The indication for palliative chemotherapy is mainly symptom control. Symptoms from SVC compression, pulmonary infiltrate, brachial plexopathy or liver disease may be controlled. If a patient has no symptoms, the use of chemotherapy is questionable. Chemotherapy may occasionally be indicated to avoid imminent symptoms, such as rapidly progressive lung lesions or early symptoms due to invasion of a nerve plexus. Prolongation of life may be the hope, but it is not often achieved, except in small cell lung cancer and ovarian cancer, when a small but significant extension of survival may be achieved. Patients taking chemotherapy deserve optimism from their professional carers that it will be effective. FBC should be checked before each dose.

Duration of chemotherapy treatment is usually 3-6 months, but the optimum length of treatment is not known. If there is evidence of progression of the disease after 6 weeks, treatment is usually stopped. On the other hand if the disease is responding and symptoms have been controlled and the patient is tolerating the chemotherapy well, it may justify extending the treatment programme.

Side-effects of chemotherapy (and usual time of onset after treatment):

- Nausea and vomiting (1-2 days)
- Marrow suppression* (7-10 days)
- Malaise (7-14 days)
- Mucositis (7-14 days)
- Hair loss, reversible (7-21days)
- neuropathy (weeks)
- lung fibrosis (weeks)

* Vincristine and Bleomycin are unusual in causing no marrow suppression.

SIDE EFFECTS OF THE COMMON CYTOTOXICS

Aclarubicin	-	see doxorubicin
Carboplatin	-	marrow, nausea (other side-effects occur less than with cisplatin)
Chlorambucil	-	marrow
Cisplatin	-	marrow, nausea, renal damage, peripheral neuropathy, high tone deafness
Cyclophosphamide	-	haemorhagic cystitis (use Mesna)
Dacarbazine	-	marrow, nausea (severe)
Etoposide	-	marrow, nausea, alopecia
Doxorubicin	-	marrow, nausea, hair loss, mucositis, cardiotoxic
Fluoruracil	-	marrow, rash (rare cerebellar syndrome)
Ifosphamide	-	haemorrhagic cystitis (use Mesna)
Lomustine	-	marrow (delayed 4-6 weeks), nausea
Melphalan	-	marrow (delayed 4-6 weeks)
Mitomycin	-	marrow (delayed 4-6 weeks), renal damage, lung fibrosis
Mitozantrone	-	marrow, cardiotoxic
Procarbazine	-	marrow, nausea, rash
Vinblastine	-	marrow
Vincristine	-	alopecia, neuropathy
Vindesine	-	marrow (less risk of neuropathy than vincristine)

Starting chemotherapy in far-advanced disease is usually illogical, but occasionally it is helpful. Some patients cope better, psychologically, by knowing they are still having treatment aimed at controlling the cancer, and will request chemotherapy treatment, even when the chances of response

CYTOTOXICS THAT CAUSE VOMITING

Cisplatin
Dacarbazine
Cyclophosphamide
Lomustine
Carboplatin
Doxorubicin
Daunorubicin
Cytarabine
Procarbazine
Etoposide
Mitomycin-C
Methotrexate
Flurouracil
Hydroxyurea
Bleomycin
Vinblastine
Vincristine
Vindesine
Chlorambucil

(Nausea and vomiting is severe with drugs at the top of this list, and rare with drugs at the bottom of the list.)

are known to be very poor. It is obviously important that the doctor clearly explains the true position and that an agent is only given if it is known to be occasionally helpful (such as chlorambucil in cancer of the ovary, or 5FU in gastro-intestinal cancers). It should be given in doses that avoid side-effects.

Stopping Chemotherapy can present a dilemma. If the disease progresses despite chemotherapy it should be stopped, but there is often the fear that it may upset the patient by removing hope. The key question is: "Does the chemotherapy make you feel better?". If the patient feels better, either physically or psychologically, the chemotherapy should usually be continued. However, if it is making the patient feel worse, it is time to rest from the chemotherapy and to focus on symptom control and quality of remaining life. There comes a point when it can be a great relief for a patient and family to discuss this and to stop unhelpful treatment.

Chemotherapy in individual cancers is discussed in the separate sections on cancers.

References:
Rubens RD *et al.* Appropriate chemotherapy for palliating advanced cancer. BMJ 1992; 304:35-40 (4.1.92)
Rakovsky E et al, 5-Fluorouracil and high dose folinic acid in symptomatic advanced colorectal carcinona; importance of symptomatic relief. Palliative Medicine 1991; 5: 250-255.

COLON CANCER

Cancer of the colon causes about 13,000 deaths per year in the UK. It is more common with a history of familial polyposis, recurrent polyps or longstanding ulcerative colitis.

Presentation of cancer of the colon is typically with altered bowel habit (diarrhoea or constipation). Lesions in the ascending or transverse colon may present with weight loss and anaemia, lesions in the descending or sigmoid colon are more likely to cause blood-stained diarrhoea or obstruction and colic.

Diagnosis is by colonoscopy and barium enema. Only 10% have a palpable abdominal mass. 10% are missed on barium enema alone.

Treatment of colonic cancer is surgical, and involves resection of the segment of colon involved (together with the lymph nodes draining it) and re-anastomosis. The cancer may involve adjacent bowel, stomach or abdominal wall, when multiple organ resection may be needed (and can still result in cure). Resection may not be possible if there is obstruction or perforation, when a temporary, defunctioning loop colostomy can be performed to improve the patient's condition prior to resection at a later date (if the patient is well enough) after which the colostomy can be reversed. Even with metastases, resection of the tumour may still offer the best form of palliation.

Metastases from colonic cancer occur in the liver, and less commonly to bone, lung or brain. Liver metastases can be resected if there are only up to 3 discrete metastases, with an 80% 1 year survival rate. (Ultrasound cutting devices are often used for resection). Other methods of treating hepatic metastases include laser, alcohol injection, interstitial radiotherapy, cryotherapy and localized chemotherapy via the hepatic artery (Gut 1993; 34: 1156–7).

Prognosis depends on how far the cancer has spread through the mucosa. 5 year survival is 90% if the disease is confined to the mucosa (Duke's stage A), falling to 60% if it has spread through the mucosa (Duke's B) and 25% if lymph nodes are involved (Duke's C).

Chemotherapy with intravenous fluorouracil with folinic acid (which potentiates the effect of fluorouracil) give the best response rates, of around 20%. Chemotherapy is only indicated to improve symptoms. Treatment is monitored clinically and by chest X-ray and liver ultrasound, and continues for 4-6 cycles if a response occurs. Continuous infusions have no advantages over intermittent injections. Intrahepatic arterial infusion of 5FU has been disappointing and should be considered a research technique. Other cytotoxics (lomustine, mitomycin) have been used but offer no advantages over fluorouracil.

A study of 16 patients with colo-rectal tumours showed that fluorouracil and folinic acid improved symptoms (pain, anorexia and malaise) in 9 patients (60%) for 2-14 months (median 6.5 months), even though only 4 showed any objective regression (Rakowsky, Palliative Medicine 1991; 5: 250-55).

Problems of advanced cancer of the colon include:

- Pain
- Ascites
- Intestinal obstruction
- Abdominal fistula

COMPLEMENTARY THERAPIES

Complementary therapies offer an individualized and personal approach to illness and can greatly improve a patient's quality of life. In a survey at Hammersmith hospital, 60% of cancer patients said they wanted to try complementary therapies. There is no evidence that they control tumour growth or improve prognosis.

Patients with advanced disease are often searching for comfort more than cure. Even when a person has accepted that their illness is incurable, it is still a reasonable goal to search for ways to feel better rather than necessarily to get better. There are many different therapies around, but they share certain characteristics in what they offer:

- Time and attention
- Listening
- Touching
- Authority\charisma
- Hope of improvement

Two particular problems can arise with some practitioners of complementary therapies. They may make unrealistic claims of cure and may charge high prices. Provided cure is not being claimed most complementary therapies can be encouraged.

Complementary therapies discussed here include:

- Special diets
- Vitamins and Minerals
- Homeopathy
- Acupuncture
- Stress reduction techniques
  - Massage
  - Aromatherapy
  - Visualization
  - Muscular relaxation

- Biofeedback
- Breathing exercises
- Meditation
- Reflexology
- Faith Healing
- Hypnosis
- Art therapy\Music therapy
- Other techniques, including:
  - Shiatsu
  - Kinesiology (Touch for Health)
  - Iridology

Special diets tend to be high in fibre and raw foods and fruit, low in sugar and salt, and are usually vegetarian, including vegetable and fruit juices. They are partly based on the assumption that since a poor diet may help cause cancer, a good diet *may* retard or cure cancer. Macrobiotic (meaning "great life") diets stress the effect of healthy eating on quality of life, and promote foods which are whole, locally grown and seasonally fresh.

There is no evidence that diet affects established cancer. There is epidemiological evidence that a high fibre diet lowers the incidence of bowel cancer in a population. Fibre is known to bind some carcinogens (cancer-forming residues) and the Western diet includes some substances such as mycotoxins and nitrosamines which have been implicated as cancer-promoting in some experimental animals.

Vitamins and minerals remain popular, and some patients take large quantities of complex and often expensive combinations, in the hope of feeling better or prolonging their life. There is little evidence that they have any influence on the cancer.

Vitamin C, vitamin E, retinoids and flavinoids may protect against experimental cancer in some animals. There is no evidence that they have any effects on established cancer. However, they are harmless, in the correct doses, and if no extravagant claims have been made for them, they can be gently encouraged as *possibly* beneficial. Some substances however may be harmful.

Laetrile, derived from bitter almonds, was widely used in the 1970's as a cancer treatment, but a prospective controlled randomized trial in 178 patients with advanced cancer showed no regression or improvement and some patients had dangerously high cyanide levels.

Selenium is sometimes advocated for cancer patients. There is also evidence that people with very low selenium levels have double the risk of developing cancer. Selenium is an essential element in man and is a component of glutathione peroxidase which helps protect macromolecules from oxidation stress. There is some geographical evidence linking high selenium levels in soil with a reduced mortality from cancer. Some population studies have shown that low plasm selenium levels are associated with a slightly higher risk of developing cancer. There is no evidence that selenium affects the course of existing cancer.

Vitamin E (Efamol) given in a placebo-controlled trial to 25 patients with Dukes C colo-rectal cancer did not increase survival (Br Med J 1987; 294: 1260)

Homeopathy is a system of medicine which was developed in the 1850's by Samual Hahnemann, in response to the harsh and useless bleeding and purging therapies of the day. It is based on the idea that symptoms are due to an imbalance or dysharmony of the whole person, and the whole person is treated rather than the disease. The principle of homeopathy is that "like cures like", meaning that if a substance causes certain symptoms then a minute quantity of the same substance will cure those symptoms.

For example diluted extract of onion may be given for the symptoms of running eyes and stinging throat due to the common cold and diluted extract of bee sting may be given for swelling, since a bee sting causes swelling. Homeopathy involves matching the remedy to the symptoms. A detailed history of symtoms and emotional state is taken. For example there are several different remedies for nausea, depending on the type of nausea and the physical and emotional state of the patient. The principle is that one substance is tried at a time. Injections of iscador (derived from mistletoe) are sometimes prescribed for cancer patients. Homeopathic remedies have the great advantage that they do not cause side-effects, and this is because the remedies contain no active ingredients. They are derived from the original substances by a system of dilutions and shakings ("sucussions") until there is none of the original substance left. This makes it hard to explain how they can possibly work, but there is no shortage of anecdotes to support the effectiveness of homeopathic remedies for a wide variety of symptoms. There are no comparative studies which suggest that they are effective.

Acupuncture is mainly used to relieve pain in a variety of non-malignant conditions such as arthritis and migraine. The shorter the duration of the pain, the better the response. The mechanism of pain relief is probably the release of endogenous opioids. An early study showed that the CSF from a rabbit receiving acupuncture, injected into the brain of another rabbit, will raise its pain threshold. Traditional Chinese acupuncture, practised for over 4000 years, is based on the theory that needle insertions alter the flow of energy along certain meridians of the body, restoring the balance of the forces (Yin and Yang) in the body. Western practitioners tend to use the theory of focal points, and may use electrical or laser stimulation instead of needles. Acupuncture can reduce dyspnoea due to COAD (Lancet 1986; ii:1416-20) and may be able to reduce some types of vomiting (Lancet 1987; i: 1083).

Massage combines physical relaxation with therapeutic touch, and reduces stress both by reducing muscular tension and by reducing feelings of isolation. Many patients regress and need more physical touch. Essential oils can enhance the effects of massage (*see Aromatherapy*). Massage also conveys empathy and encourages trust and the ventilation of feelings.

6 different types of hand movement are involved:

- Effleurage (gentle stroking)
- Petrissage (squeezing)
- Tapotement (fine quick vibratory movements)
- Kneading (firm stroking)
- Hacking (firm tapping with the edges of both hands)
- Cupping (like hacking, but using cupped hands)

Aromatherapy uses essential oils, sometimes with massage, to achieve deep relaxation. Frankincense, camomile, lavender and vetivert are all said to calming and soothing. Hippocrates wrote "The way to health is to have a scented bath and an oiled massage each day". The sense of smell can powerfully affect emotions and memories. Touch and smell are both primitive senses and massage with aromatic oils can induce deep relaxation. Some of the essential oils may be absorbed transdermally in minute quantities (camomile, basil). Aromatherapists may also recommend the use of inhalations, bath oils and lotions.

Visualization is the regular imagining of a desired outcome (such as shrinkage of the tumour). It is practised 2-3 times a day for 15-20 minutes, and encourages a patient to develop a feeling of control. The patient pictures the cancer (in whatever form they choose) as weak and confused and the body's defences as strong. Visualization is intended to reduce the feelings of helplessness, which lead to depression. Discussion of the patient's imagary may reveal fears or misconceptions about treatment. Cancer treatments should be seen as promoting the body's defences. There is some evidence that regular visualization can improve some parameters of the immune system. The technique is described in detail in the book "Getting Well Again" by Simonton OC, Mathews-Simonton S and Creighton JL, Bantam Books.

Muscular relaxation, contracting and relaxing different groups of muscles, according to instructions from a therapist (or a tape) is a useful method of inducing a certain amount of relaxation, and is a useful starting point for patients finding it difficult to begin to relax mentally.

Biofeedback measures physiological parameters in order to teach the patient to recognize when they are becoming more relaxed. It measures pulse rate, skin resistance (sweating) and electro-myography (muscle tension).

Breathing exercises can be especially useful if the patient is tending to hyperventilate. They focus on full expiration, lowering the shoulders and using the diaphragm when inhaling (so the abdomen rises). It is often very helpful to teach the relatives as well, so they know what to encourage in times of panic.

Meditation is a method of reducing the arousal level by means of focused attention using:

- A visual image
- A repeated sound
- Physical repetition (breathing)

If meditation is practised regularly it can induce deep relaxation. It demands mental concentration and may be impossible if the patient is tense, when a more basic program of relaxation may be needed first.

Reflexology is massage of the feet. It is based on the theory that there are 10 zones of energy flow, running the length of the body, and that foot massage can remove congestion and energy blocks from the pathways, and normalize the function of internal organs. There is no evidence that this occurs, but many patients find it relaxing.

Faith Healing includes a variety of approaches, often combining touch, positive thinking and listening (sometimes in a religious context) and it usually also results in deep relaxation.

Hypnosis can be defined as an altered state of consciousness, characterized by change in mood, sensation, perception and memory, which allows greater access to unconscious processes. There is diminished critical awareness and selective attention. It could be described as "assisted meditation". Suggestibility is enhanced, which can be used to program muscular relaxation or analgesia. There is also an increased capacity for role enactment ("as if" feelings) which can be maintained by post-hypnotic suggestion. It can result in deep relaxation and can reduce fears. It is also used to increase feelings of self-control. Glove and stocking anaesthesia can be induced by a variety of suggestions directed at localizing physical sensations. This ability to control sensation of pain can sometimes be used to demonstrate control of and reduced awareness of physical pain.

Art therapy\Music therapy and other creative diversional therapies can reduce stress levels, provide a sense of purpose and improve self-esteem (see *Spiritual support*).

Further reading:
Rankin-Box DF, Editor, Complementary Health Therapies: A Guide for Nurses and the Caring Professions, 1988, Croom Helm Ltd.
Sims S. The significance of touch in palliative care. Palliative Medicine 1988; 2: 58-61.
Willett WC, Stampfer MJ, Selenium and Cancer, Br Med J, 3 Sept 1988; 297: 573-4).
Filshie J, Morrison PJ. Acupuncture for chronic pain: a review. Palliative Medicine 1988; 2: 1-14.

CONFUSION

Confusion (or delirium) means a toxic confusional state due to an organic cause, characterized by *decreased attention* and *cognitive* *impairment.* If no specific cause can be found, it is assumed that the delirium is due to advancing malignant disease or a para-neoplastic syndrome. It is made worse by deafness.

Prevalence of confusion depends on the population of patients studied, and the sensitivity of the tests used to detect it, from 8% (for all stages of cancer, inpatient and outpatient) to 25-40% (for all stages of cancer, inpatients only) to as high as 85% for hospitalized terminally ill patients. It is particularly common in elderly patients who are moved from a familiar environment.

Diagnosis of confusion may be obvious, with altered or inappropriate behaviour (agitated *or* withdrawn), and incoherent, rambling speech. The clinical picture is sometimes described as "clouded consciousness". The typical features are:

- Rapid onset (hours or days)
- Reduced awareness (of the environment)
- Drowsiness (yet easily startled)
- Poor concentration
- Poor short-term memory
- Disorientation (for time, place or person)

The patient may appear drowsy, with a reduced awareness of the environment and yet is easily startled. It often fluctuates (worse in the evenings) with lucid intervals of normal intellectual function (when a will can be legally signed). The patient may have insight into the confusion ("I am not myself at the moment").

Severe confusion can progress to psychotic features, with delusions (illogical beliefs, especially related to being harmed) and hallucinations (visual and auditory). Rarely, one feature may dominate the clinical picture, with:

- Impaired memory (organic amnesic syndrome)
- Delusions (organic delusional syndrome)
- Hallucinations (organic hallucinosis)
- Change in mood (organic affective syndrome)

The correct management of confusion brings relief even when confusion cannot be reversed. It involves:

- Control of the situation
- Look for reversible causes
- Regulate the environment
- Understand fears
- Consider sedation

Control of the situation is the first step. Delirium is frightening to the patient and relatives. It is the most difficult symptom to cope with in the home. A calm and trusted person should listen to fears and explain ("You are not going mad, this is part of your illness"). Even a very agitated patient will respond to a quiet environment, explanation and reassurance. Sedation is only necessary if the patient may harm themselves or others. Try to persuade the patient to take something "to calm the nerves" (*see below*). Restraint, if the patient is violent, requires 3 professional carers. It is best to manoeuvre the patient (preferably by verbal persuasion) onto a bed and into the lateral position, and give an IM injection of Chlorpromazine 100mg with hyoscine 0.4mg.

Exclude reversible causes (discussed in more detail below) especially:

- Pain (full bladder or impaction?)
- Drugs
- Injury (Subdural haematoma – CT scan)
- Brain metastases
- Heart failure (?infarct)
- Hypoxia (pulse oximeter)
- Infection (urine, chest)
- Biochemical (U&E, LFTs, calcium, glucose)
- Withdrawals (alcohol, benzodiazepines)
- Extreme anxiety

Regulation of the environment, means a quiet, well-lit room, with a few familiar people (staff and relatives). Avoid sudden changes. Explain all proceedures. A large wall clock should be easily visible. Take opportunities to orientate the patient ("It is Monday morning", "I am the doctor. I expect you remember our talk yesterday about your wife").

Fear is a typical feature of confusion. Often the patient has insight: ("I am not myself at the moment"). The patient has difficulty separating internal thoughts and external events. Understanding this can help: ("No, I am not your mother, but I can understand your feelings, and I imagine you wish I was your mother"). Fears relating to previous experiences can re-surface. Help the person to distinguish past from present. The patient may feel threatened ("they are killing me with these drugs") – and may need explanation from a trusted person the illness is due to the disease not the surroundings.

Sedation will not reverse confusion, but may be necessary if the patient is not accessible to counselling. Haloperidol 3-10mg BD is helpful if there is a psychotic element, with abnormal behaviour or experiences (paranoia, hallucinations, delusions). Haloperidol 10mg orally usually takes about an hour to take effect. The solution for injection can be given orally, and is tasteless. Lorazepam 1-2mg orally, or a continuous subcutaneous infusion of Midazolam 20-40mg, may be sufficient if anxiety is the main problem and there is no altered behaviour or abnormal experiences. Chlorpromazine 10-75mg QID is more sedating, but is useful if agitation or restlessness are the main features (start with a low dose, as it is very sedating for some patients). An anti-depressant such as amitriptyline or dothiepin, 10-25mg TID may be indicated for an agitated depression. Lorazepam 0.5-1mg BD can be useful if anxiety or panic are the main features.

Causes of confusion:

Drugs that can cause confusion include phenothiazines, tricyclics, benzodiazepines, cimetidine, phenytoin, pentazocine, indomethacin, digoxin, beta-blockers, diuretics, sulphonamides, benzhexol. N.B. Doses that have been tolerated for months may suddenly become toxic (because renal and hepatic function can deteriorate as malignant disease progresses). Anti-cholinergic delerium (fever, flushing, widely dilated pupils, tachycardia, sometimes urinary retention) can occur if anti-cholinergic drugs (cyclizine, phenothiazines, tricyclics, anti-spasmodics, anti-Parkinsonian drugs) are used together. Steroids can cause restlessness and insomnia, which can progress to agitation and delerium, most likely to occur when first started or if the dose is increased. Morphine only causes confusion if the dose is poorly balanced. Confusion is avoided if the dose is decreased whenever the patient is painfree and drowsy.

Brain metastases can cause delerium, usually with obvious neurological signs. The diagnosis can be confirmed by CT scan, but if the patient is not well enough to have a scan, a trial of high dose steroids (dexamethasone 16mg a day) is indicated.

Myocardial infarct may be silent (with no chest pain) and present as sudden confusion. There may be left ventricular failure. CVA may also cause sudden confusion, and the diagnosis may not be obvious if the limbs and speech are unaffected.

Hypoxia is suspected from tachycardia, cyanosis and restlessness, and confimed by a blood gas or, less invasively, by a pulse oximeter. Oxygen will help if the patient is hypoxic.

Infection (fever, sweats, flushing, tachycardia) may be masked by steroids, so always send a MSU for culture, and consider a chest Xray and blood cultures (lumbar puncture is rarely indicated).

Biochemical causes (hyponatraemia, uraemia, hypercalcaemia and diabetes) can all present with (or can worsen) confusion. Even when there is no treatment, as with uraemia, it is still very helpful to know the reason for confusion, so that explanation can be given and other causes do not need to be pursued (see Hypercalcaemia and Diabetes).

Hyponatraemia (plasma sodium below 120 mmol\l) is a rare cause of confusion, and can be occur with SIADH (see Ectopic hormones).

Extreme anxiety can cause confusion, as an emotional defense against fear. It can improve if the patient begins to feel more secure. Such patients can benefit greatly from formal psychotherapy, often using cognitive approaches.

Alcohol withdrawal can cause delerium tremens (confusion, tremor, sweats, hallucinations, seizures) which may not develop for several days (see Alcohol).

Mental testing can detect intellectual impairment in confusion, which causes a reversible inability to take in new information. The following simple test (see table) can be useful, a score under 10 indicating significant intellectual impairment.

SIMPLIFIED MENTAL TEST SCORE

Ask: "Do you mind if I test your memory?"

Question	Possible Score
● What is the date today? (day, month, year)	3
● What is the address here? (3 parts)	3
● I am going to test you with numbers- can you take 7 away from 100? Again? Again? ("Serial sevens" 93,86,79,72,65 then stop)	5
● Can you tell me what this is called? (choose 3 simple objects such as a watch, a glass and a pencil).	3
● Name 3 imagined objects and ask the patient to remember and recall them (after the next task)	3
● I want you to take the paper in your right hand, fold it and place it on the table (3-stage command)	3
TOTAL SCORE:	20

Score of 10 or less indicates significant intellectual impairment.

Further reading:
Fleishman S, Lesko LM, Delerium and Dementia, in Holland JC and Rowland JH (Eds), Handbook of Psycho-oncology, Oxford University Press, Oxford 1989.
Stedeford A, Facing Death: Patients, Families and Professionals. London, Heinemann Medical Books, 1984.
Folstein MF, Folstein SE, McHugh PR, "Mini-mental state", a practical method for grading the cognitive state of patients for the clinician. J Psychiat. Res, 1975, Vol 12: 189-198.

CONSTIPATION

Constipation means hard or infrequent motions. 50% of hospice patients are constipated on admission, even though many have been taking laxatives (but incorrectly).

Causes of constipation include poor diet, dehydration, diuretics and anti-cholinergics, but opioids are the commonest cause of severe constipation. The following patients need laxatives:

- 90% on morphine
- 70% on co-proxamol
- 40% not on analgesics

Morphine causes constipation in most patients, unless they have malabsorbtion due to steatorrhoea or a small bowel resection). Opioids increase the ring contractions in the colon (which normally serve to mix bowel contents) and this slows forward movement of stools and increases water absorbtion, making stools harder.

The symptoms of constipation can include:

- Abdominal discomfort
- Malaise
- Anorexia
- Nausea and vomiting
- Colic
- Impaction, tenesmus
- Faecal incontinence
- Urinary retention
- Obstruction
- Mental confusion

The signs of constipation are indentable lumps in the left side of the abdomen, (and faecal masses indent and move with time, whereas tumour masses do not) and hard faeces palpable on rectal examination. The rectum may be empty and ballooned in high constipation. Abdominal Xray shows faeces (and not gas or fluid levels).

Impacted faeces can be diagnosed from the history (although the patient may be too embarrassed to give it) of:

- Prolonged constipation (7-21 days)
- Chipping out faeces with a finger
- Small liquid faeces
- Faecal leak
- Pain (colic, tenesmus or both)

Digital removal of the impacted faeces may be necessary. It should be performed under heavy sedation. A useful method is an I.M. injection of diamorphine (dose=half 4 hourly oral morphine dose) with chlorpromazine 25mg and hyoscine 0.4mg. Alternatively I.V. midazolam 1–5mg by slow injection is useful. In the rare event of respiratory depression midazolam can be reversed by I.V. flumazenil.

Prevention of constipation should be aggressive. High fibre diets are not well tolerated and most patients need laxatives. The principles of prevention are:

- Laxatives with all opioids
- Daily increase in dose
- The 3 day rule

The aim of laxative treatment is ease of defaecation, not a particular bowel frequency, but it is sensible to use a suppository or micro-enema if the bowels have not been open for 3 days. Improving a patient's independence can sometimes prevent constipation (raised toilet seat, hand rails).

Laxatives are needed by the majority of patients with advanced cancer. All patients on opioids need a faecal softener plus a stimulant laxative, taken daily. The aim of laxative treatment is ease of defaecation (not a particular stool frequency). It often takes several days to regulate the bowels with laxatives. The dose is titrated to response. Unfortunately no laxative is universally acceptable and alternatives are needed (*see Laxatives*).

Rectal agents (enemas and suppositories) are needed when laxatives fail or are not tolerated. Rectal agents are mainly softeners, but also have some local stimulant action. If there is no bowel movement for 3 days on laxatives use:

- Glycerol suppository, with
- Bisacodyl suppository (5mg), or
- Citrate micro-enema (5ml)

Bisacodyl is a stimulant, and acts within one hour. It is useful in "soft impaction" when the rectum is full of soft faeces but fails to empty. For more severe constipation use:

- Arachis oil enema (130ml)
- Phosphate enema (130ml)

Oil enemas soften the motions and should be retained as long as possible, and is then followed by the phosphate enema which stimulates peristalsis. Magnesium sulphate is a useful additional measure for constipation that is proving resistant to high doses of laxatives and rectal measures. 10-20ml in the morning, taken with plenty of water usually starts to cause diarrhoea 3-6 hours later (*see Laxatives*).

Anal fissure is a complication of constipation, and can cause severe pain on defaecation, with a dull ache for some hours after. The fissure is usually posterior, sometimes with a sentinel skin tag visible ("pile") and spasm of the sphincter. Treatment options are:

- Lignocaine gel before defaecation
- Bulking agent to soften stool (Fybogel BD)
- Surgical referral to consider:
  - Dilatation of the anus
  - Subcutaneous sphincterotomy

Normal defaecation varies from twice a day to twice a week. transit time through the bowel varies from 1-5 days, and 90% of that transit time occurs in the colon.

The colon's function is to absorb water from the stools, which normally contain about 75% water. Colonic delay increases stool hardness, allowing more water to be absorbed. Constipated stools only contain about 60% water.

The rectum acts as a reservoir for faeces, until it is socially acceptable to defaecate. It is normally empty, until a forward peristalsis of the colon (a mass movement) occurs (1-2 times a day). A bowel movement normally consists of the contents of the rectum only, but with stimulant laxatives can be from the whole colon. Rectal stenosis caused by pelvic tumours can cause difficulty in defaecating, or tenesmus (or both).

N.B. Patients eating little continue to produce waste in the bowel (gut secretions, desquamation, and bacteria) and can still become constipated.

COUGH

Productive cough, with sputum, may be due to a chest infection, lung abscess, heart failure or bronchitis. Rarely, an alveolar cell carcinoma of the lung can produce large volumes of clear, watery sputum (bronchorrhoea).

Treatment options for a productive cough include:

- Antibiotics
- Diuretics
- Physiotherapy
- Nebulized saline\steam inhalations

Green infective sputum should normally be treated with a broad-spectrum antibiotic such as Augmentin, after sending some sputum for culture. Metronidazole (Flagyl) 400mg TID will reduce smell from a lung abscess. White frothy sputum suggests left ventricular failure (LVF). Other features are orthopnoea, tachycardia, basal crepitations and a third heart sound. The symptoms respond to a diuretic, frusemide 40-80mg daily. Physiotherapy (gentle percussion with forced expiration) can help loosen sputum and allow expectoration. Patients are usually too weak for postural drainage, and physiotherapy needs to be performed carefully, because in ill patients vigourous therapy may cause bronchospasm or transient hypoxia. Nebulized saline\steam inhalations can both help loosen tenacious sputum. There is no evidence that expectorants (such as ammonium chloride) or mucolytics (such as acetylycysteine or carbocysteine) are effective.

Dry cough can be more difficult to treat. It may be due a bronchial tumour mass, multiple lung secondaries, bronchospasm or a pleural effusion. It can cause:

- Insomnia
- Exhaustion
- Vomiting
- Rib fracture ("cough fracture")
- Cough syncope

Treatment options for a dry cough include:

- Radiotherapy
- Antitussives (codeine, morphine, methadone)
- Steroids
- Bronchodilators
- Nebulized local anaesthetic
- Interpleural local anaesthetic

Radiotherapy can be helpful when a cough is due to irritation from a large bronchial tumour, especially a hilar tumour involving the bifurcation of the bronchi. Palliative radiotherapy to a bronchial tumour will reduce cough in about 40% of cases.

Antitussives. The strongest antitussive is morphine. Codeine is probably effective because it is metabolized to morphine. Methadone linctus (2mg in 5ml) 5-10ml nocte or TID, will sometimes help to control a dry cough when morphine does not, and can be helpful in a patient already on morphine (for unknown reasons). (Dextromethorphan is a mild non-opioid antitussive that is an ingredient in many commercial compound cough preparations).

Steroids in high doses (dexamethasone 6-12mg daily) can help to reduce a dry cough due to a bronchial mass, lung metastases or reversible airways obstruction (*see Steroids*).

Bronchodilators will abolish cough that is due to bronchospasm. Late-onset asthma is very common, and should always be considered in cases of persistent dry cough. A peak flow meter is useful to monitor the response to bronchodilator treatment, which may include:

- Nebulized salbutamol
- Nebulized ipratropium
- Theophyllines

Salbutamol (Ventolin) nebulizer solution, 2.5-5mg, 2-4 hourly, is often effective. High doses can cause a marked tremor, when the dose should be reduced and other bronchodilators used in addition.

Ipratropium (Atrovent) is available as nebulizer solution, 250 micrograms per ml. Nebules can be diluted with normal saline, usually to 5 ml, prior to use in the nebulizer. Dose is 250-500 micrograms 4 hourly.

Salbutamol and ipratropium act in different ways and can be logically combined in the same mixture for severe wheeze, but used together may rarely precipitate acute glaucoma (eye pain, blurred vision) in susceptible patients (those who are long-sighted with a shallow anterior chamber to the eye). This is due to the nebulized mist of drugs escaping from the mask and acting directly on the eye. Emergency treatment involves 4% pilocarpine drops, 500mg acetazolamide IV and analgesia.

Slow-release Theophyllines (e.g. Slo-phyllin 250-500mg BD or Phylocontin 225-450mg BD) can both reverse airways obstruction, and can be very useful for patients who cannot manage inhalers, or are already receiving inhaled or nebulized medication and need additional bronchodilation. They can be especially useful for night cough, as a single dose at bedtime. The dose should be started low and increased after a week, to avoid side-effects (mainly nausea). They have a narrow therapeutic range and alterations in metabolism can be clinically significant. Higher doses are needed with phenytoin or carbamazepine. Lower doses are needed with cimetidine, erythromycin or ciprofloxacin.

Nebulized local anaesthetic. Nebulized 2% lignocaine or 0.5% bupivacaine, 5ml 4 hourly, will reduce cough that is due to distortion of the larger bronchi by a lung cancer or lung metastases. The effect is occasionally dramatic. Pharygeal numbness may occur, so the patient must be advised not to eat or drink anything (other than plain water) for 30 minutes after treatment. It can worsen bronchospasm, and is contra-indicated if there is a history of asthma.

Inhaled drugs reach the lungs in varying proportions, depending on the method of administration: Nebulized drugs reach the lungs most efficiently and are easier to use for weak patients:

- Inhaler (11%)
- Space inhaler (17%)
- Nebuhaler (30%)
- Nebulizer (35%)

Intrapleural local anaesthetic infusion can be considered for intractable cough that is not controlled by other methods. An epidural catheter can be placed in the pleural space, on the side of the lung disease, and 20ml of 0.5% bupivacaine infused 12 hourly. This can be very effective in controlling both chest wall pain and also cough, (possibly by blocking vagal fibres, which carry the sensory messages of the cough reflex to the medulla).

ACE inhibitors (Angiotensin-converting-enzyme inhibitors) used in the treatment of hypertension, can cause a persistent dry cough as a side-effect. They include captopril (Capoten) and enalapril (Innovace).

Terminal coughing is best controlled with morphine and an anti-cholinergic to dry up secretions. Hyoscine 0.4mg 4 hourly is effective and sedating. Atropine 0.6mg 4 hourly can be useful if the patient does not want to be sedated or drowsy. Suction is only occasionally helpful if the patient is distressed by tenacious sputum at the back of the throat, but repeated suction is distressing and should be avoided.

COUNSELLING

Counselling can be defined as therapeutic listening, which encourages the expression of feelings and increased self-confidence. 50% of hospice patients and families actively seek counselling help for their emotions.

The aim of counselling is to provide an opportunity for change (of assumptions, thoughts, feelings, attitudes or behaviour). The counsellor must avoid the temptation to force the rate or direction of that change. It is important to make a formal contract, agreeing at the outset how long and how often the sessions are to last.

6 types of counselling intervention have been described (Heron, 1986) which encompass all possible types of intervention. This list is very useful when considering ones own repertoir of techniques as a counsellor. The types of intervention are:

1. Prescriptive
2. Informative
3. Confronting
4. Cathartic
5. Catalytic
6. Supportive

The first three are authoritative, the second three are facilitative. Many counsellors feel least skilled at the confronting and cathartic interventions.

1. Prescriptive interventions start "I would recommend that...". This type of intervention can occasionally be helpful in reducing uncertainty in a situation calling for clear leadership, but over-used it becomes heavy-handed and can increase a person's dependence on the counsellor, which is the opposite intention to that of good counselling.

2. Informative interventions impart knowledge or information, which must be appropriate to the person's needs. Never give unrequested information, especially bad news, which simply causes anxiety and denial. Ideally the information involves concrete facts that reduce anxiety and clarify the person's choices, to help them make informed decisions. Avoid the temptation of passing opinions on a person's life situation or emotions (even when asked to do so). This is rarely helpful and may seem patronizing (see Explanation).

3. Confronting interventions are where emotionally-charged observations are fed back to the person. This has to be done gently because a description can feel like a criticism or judgement. The observation needs to be sandwiched between an affirmation of the person and some subsequent follow-up support. The affirmation may simply be non-verbal, such as eye contact with a smile. The observation should be stated quietly and calmly and if necessary repeatedly. It can feel risky for the counsellor, because of the emotions involved, and there is a temptation to hide ones own anxiety by over-talking or being too brief and aggressive. The observations may be about behaviour (e.g. "I noticed that you seemed to change the subject when I mentioned your husband") or about negative attitudes (e.g. "You often seem to assume that you have no control over the situation") or about the counsellor's own emotions (e.g. "I am feeling quite helpless and hopeless at the moment"). The follow-up phase of support may involve a comment like "How does that make you feel" and allowing time for the person to think about their feelings.

4. Cathartic interventions allow the person to express emotions and release their pent-up tension. The main emotions relate to basic human needs and are often associated with certain behaviour (see table).

EMOTION	BASIC HUMAN NEED	BEHAVIOUR
Anger	Loss of choice	Loudness of the voice
Fear	Loss of knowing what is happening	Restlessness
Grief	Loss of love	Tears
Shame	Loss of self-respect	Embarrassed Laughter

Pent-up emotions can cause a variety of problems: muscular tension, loss of concentration, feelings of confusion, low self-esteem, misery, inappropriate behaviour, distorted attitudes, overwork or setting impossible goals (to distract from the emotional turmoil).

Encouraging the expression of emotions should only be used when the person clearly wants to do so. One method is to give permission (not to force) with a comment like "It's OK with me if you want to cry". Encouraging a description of the events associated with the feeling is often the best method, eg:

- "Tell me what happened"
- "Can you give me an example?"

Relating the feeling to physical sensations "Where in your body do you feel this", or the empty chair technique may help: "If your frustration were sitting in that chair what would you say to it?"

Emotional release is self-limiting. After it subsides the person needs time to think about the insights they gain from it. There is a link between how much emotion we, as counsellors, can allow a person to express and how much we can tolerate our own emotions, and the effective counsellor will therefore have undertaken a period of self-awareness training. Cathartic interventions tend to be exhausting and if undertaken regularly the counsellor will need a system of support (i.e. someone to listen to their feelings for a change!).

5. Catalytic (exploring) interventions often involve open questions (beginning How? What? or Why?) which open up communication of feelings. This explorative approach is essential both in routine assessment and before offering explanation. It allows a person to express needs and allows a counsellor to discover the appropriate amount of information to impart. Examples of explorative questions that can be helpful at times are:

- What has been the most difficult part of this illness for you?
- How has this illness affected your life\family\children\relationship(s)?
- What do you do to keep your spirits up?
- What would you be doing now if you were suddenly well again?
- How did you feel about coming into the hospital/hospice.
- Have you known anyone else with cancer?
- Have you felt like this before?
- What is the worst thing that could happen?
- Do you mind talking while you cry?
- What made you cry just now?
- What have you been told about your illness?
- How do you see the future?
- How long are you hoping for?
- If the time comes for you to need more nursing help, or to die, where would you like to be looked after? Why?

Reflective listening can be used to pinpoint an important emotional issues by noticing and repeating important words and phrases, which often leads to the original source of emotional distress (a process called "tracking"). Comments that seem at first to be out of place in a conversation are especially important to notice. Non sequiturs, comments that seem out of place, often relate to the person's unconscious thoughts and focusing on them, and asking about them, often brings important insights to light.

6. Supportive (encouraging) interventions are the most commonly used in counselling. The honest offer of empathy ("I am trying to understand how you feel") is supportive and encouraging. Active listening (wanting to understand what the person is saying) is of itself supportive. The counsellor must be free of his or her own concerns, including theories about what is being said, or rehearsing a reply.

Patients facing illness and death tend to regress at times and need "emotional holding" and need the security of being able to express their deepest feelings without embarrassment. Dying can be frightening and opportunities for encouragement should not be missed. Encouragement means to fill with courage. Comments such as those below can often boost morale.

- You have still got your sense of humour.
- I admire the way you are coping with all this.
- You have already survived the worst.
- Look how you have coped so far.

- You are doing well at the moment.
- You are a good patient.

Sometimes patients boost our morale as carers and when this happens we should say so and express our appreciation, which narrows the gap between the dying patient and the professional.

Mimicking is a useful technique in counselling, that can facilitate the process. The posture and non-verbal cues of the person are copied by the counsellor. These include the non-verbal aspects of speech: tone, volume, rate of speech. This has the effect of conveying empathy and can increase the effectiveness of all counselling interventions.

Hospice counselling can involve all these techniques, often in a brief and emotionally-intense relationship between a professional team member and a patient or relative. The whole process is intensified by the closeness of death, which also affects the professional carers (*see Spiritual Pain*).

The effectiveness of counselling is difficult to measure and few studies have documented or measured the effects of psycho-social interventions in the hospice setting. A review of the literature suggests a quarter to a half of patients and families want or need help in dealing with their emotional needs. One controlled study (Linn 1982) of 120 terminally ill patients showed that counselling reduced depression and increased self-esteem and quality of life and also had a positive impact on family members (*see Psychological therapy; Talking with Patients*).

Family counselling is especially valuable in the context of terminal care (*see Family support*).

Further reading:
Burnard P, Therapy in Practice Series: Counselling skills for Health Professionals, Chapman and Hall, 1989.
Vachon MLS, Counselling and psychotherapy in palliative\hospice care: a review. Palliative Medicine 1988; 2: 36-50.
Cassidy S, Emotional distress in terminal cancer: discussion paper. J Roy Soc Med 1986; 79: 717-20.

CUTANEOUS MALIGNANT SPREAD

Cutaneous malignant spread occur commonly on the chest wall after local recurrence of breast cancer, and in perineal and vulval cancers. Abdominal tumours can occasionally spread through the abdominal wall. Large lesions on the skin that are disfiguring or painful can be reduced with surgery, cryotherapy or RT.

Bleeding can be controlled with topical adrenaline 1 in 1000, or 1% Alum solution, calcium alginate dressings and oral tranexamic acid. Arterial bleeding points can be controlled by embolization (*see Bleeding*).

Routine cleaning can be done with warm normal saline. Chlorhexidine is a suitable antiseptic for very dirty areas. Smell is best controlled with topical metronidazole gel. Necrotic tissue should be excised with scissors (*see Smell*).

Discharge, if heavy, suggests a sinus or fistula has formed. Use a stoma bag to collect heavy discharge. If it is urine or faeces consider bypass surgery. Use a barrier cream to protect the skin.

Dressings should be non-adherent, absorbent and protective. Pack cavities with alginate ribbon. Apply foam or other absorbent dressing if there is a lot of exudate, and hold in place with tubular elastic netting (*see Dressings*).

Painful dressings require short-term additional analgesia at the time the dressing is done. consider using Entonox (nitrous oxide plus oxygen) or sublingual dextromoramide or rarely, for severe pain, IV alfentanyl (*see Analgesics, page 14*).

Polaroid photographs can be very useful to monitor the effects of various treatment regimes.

Psycho-social probems include:

- Altered body image
- Low morale
- Social isolation (smell)
- Sexual isolation
- Clothing (?Community laundry service)
- Dirty dressings (?Community collection service)

Reference:
Saunders J, Regnard C, Management of maligant ulcers – a flow diagram. Palliative Medicine 1989; 3: 153-155.

DEAFNESS

Deafness increases social isolation and makes communication and symptom control more difficult.

Ear wax is a common cause of deafness. Ear syringing with warm water greatly improve hearing. Ear drops worsen hearing and should only be used if wax is stubborn. 5% sodium bicarbonate drops BP are very effective. The patient should lie with the affected ear uppermost after plenty of the solution has been inserted. Syringe straight afterwards.

Postaural hearing aids (worn behind the ear) have a volume setting and an on\off switch with 3 markings:

M – Microphone on
O – Off
T – Telephone induction coil

Hearing aid centres supply new batteries (mercury camera batteries) and recommend checking of the aid every 6 months. The ear mould should fit snugly and extend 5-10mm into the auditory canal. If the hearing aid is not working, check:

- Batteries (turn up volume – should squeal)
- Ear mould (wash and remove wax with wire)
- Tubing (blow through)

Body-worn hearing aids are used for more severe deafness or for patients who cannot manage the tiny controls on the post-aural aids. They can also be used with a bone conductor for patients with severe conductive deafness due to middle ear disease.

A communicator is extremely useful with some deaf patients. An ear-piece is placed over the patient's ear, and this connects to a portable amplifier. The speaker speaks into a small microphone built into the amplifier. The "Contacta" hand-held personal communicator model HH\1 is recommended. It is small and easy to use. Available from:

- TVM (Manchester LTD)
  9 Bloom St
  Salford
  Lancashire
  Tel. 061-834-2659

DEATH CERTIFICATION

Death certification was started in 1837 to provide legal proof of death and for statistics of cause of death. The doctor in attendance during the last illness has a statutory duty to give a medical certificate of cause of death, if known. The doctor states the cause of death to the best of his belief and knowledge. If the certificate mentions the words "fracture" or "cirrhosis" the registrar is obliged to refer to the coroner. If the doctor is unsure of the cause it is sensible to discuss with the coroner. The certificate is normally given to the informant (normally a relative, but may simply be the person responsible for the funeral arrangements) who has a legal duty to inform the registrar.

The statutory proceedure for the disposal of a dead body is outlined in the flow chart. It can be helpful to understand this, because many relatives worry about the formalities after death, yet may feel guilty about seeking such information. Consider asking: "Some people worry about all the formalities after someone dies – is that one of your worries?"

Registration of death should take place within 5 days of death, in the district where the death occured (or the district where the patient lived, in Scotland). The registrar has a statutory duty to report the death to the coroner if:

- No doctor treated in last illness
- Sudden or unexplained death
- Accidental death
- Suicide
- During surgery
- War pension was held
- Death in official custody
- Industrial disease suspected
  - Asbestos (mesothelioma)
  - Mineral oils\tars (skin)
  - Nickel, leather (nasal sinus)
  - Benzidine dyes (bladder)
  - PVC manufacture (liver angiosarcoma)

The coroner or his deputy is on call 24 hours a day. Most coroners are practising solicitors employed by the Local Authority. The coroner's role is to establish the cause of death, and whether it was due to natural causes. He cannot attribute blame or guilt, which is the duty of a court of law. There is no expense to the relatives if a coroners post-mortem or inquest is held, although the funeral may have to be delayed. 30% of deaths are referred to the coroner, but most cases are referred as a formality, and no further investigations are needed.

Funeral directors usually operate a 24 hour service to transfer a body to their chapel of rest, where relatives may view the body if they wish. The funeral director requires a certificate of disposal from the registrar for permission to proceed. Funeral directors should be advised if there is any risk of infection (hepatitis B, salmonella, tuberculosis or HIV). It can be helpful to the relatives to contact the funeral director as soon as the death occurs, as is the usual practise with deaths at home. It is usual to carry out the deceased's wishes concerning burial or cremation, but there is no legal obligation on the next-of-kin (or executors) to do so. The transaction with a funeral director is a business deal. Members of the National Association of Funeral Directors must give an itemized written estimate of costs. The trade of "undertaking a funeral" started about 200 years ago when some carpenters began to specialize in producing coffins.

Cremation became a legal method of disposing of a dead body in 1902. Cremation must take place on the same day as the funeral. The regulations

THE STATUTORY PROCEDURE FOR THE DISPOSAL OF A DEAD BODY

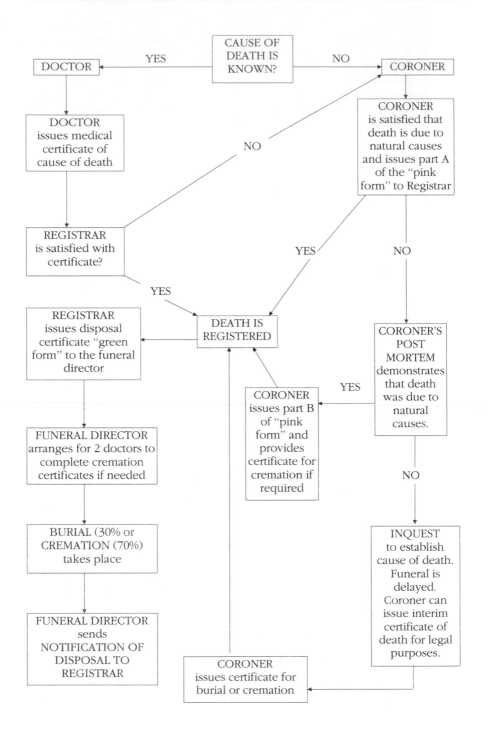

are more stringent for cremation because all traces of the body are destroyed, leaving no evidence for forensic purposes. A body can only be cremated if the cause of death is definately known. Pacemakers must be removed before cremation, as they can explode. The medical referee at the crematorium can refuse permission for a cremation and order a post-mortem. If relatives wish they can witness the commital of the body to the cremator. Most crematoria will retain the ashes, free of charge, for a month, while the relatives decide on the method of disposal, the options being to keep in an urn, bury in the crematorium or a churchyard or to scatter the ashes.

DEEP VEIN THROMBOSIS

Deep vein thrombosis (DVT) is common in terminally ill patients, because bed rest and immobility cause venous stasis. It most commonly affects the leg veins Some cancers (especially cancer of the pancreas) predispose to venous thrombosis. DVT is more common in obese patients.

Clinical features of DVT are:

- Unilateral leg swelling
- Pain
- Tenderness
- Oedema
- Cyanosis of the leg (late)
- Dilated superficial veins (late)

Tenderness can occur between the heads of gastrocnemius (where the thrombosed vein is palpable) and also in the anterior thigh, (at the saphenous opening), which suggests femoral vein thrombosis.

Pulmonary embolus causes dyspnoea (small embolus), chest pains due to pulmonary infarct (medium) or sudden death (massive). The association of DVT with pulmonary emboli is much stronger when thrombus involves the proximal leg veins, above the level of the knee.

Diagnosis of DVT is by a venogram, but can also be confirmed, if necessary, by non-invasive tests such as Doppler ultrasound or impedance plethysmography which will detect 95% of thrombi detectable on a venogram.

Management options for a DVT include:

- Analgesia and explanation
- Elastic support stocking
- Anti-coagulation
- IVC filter

Elastic support garments may relieve discomfort, but should be abandoned if uncomfortable. The aim is to provide graduated compression, with most compression at the ankle, less at the calf, and least at the thigh. Prescribe thigh-length, class 1 elastic stockings. The patient takes the prescription to the pharmacist who supplies a measurement form, for circumferences at the ankle, calf and thigh, which are best measured first thing in the morning. The stocking should be removed at night.

Anti-coagulation may be indicated to reduce severe pain and swelling in the leg or for recurrent pulmonary emboli. It normally involves IV heparin for 5 days and oral warfarin for up to 12 weeks. Anti-coagulation carries a significant risk (5-8%) of a major haemorrhage. The treatment is monitored by clotting tests. APTT is not routinely measured, but can be used to monitor heparin (aim: 1.5-2.5). The international normalized ratio (INR) is the equivalent of the prothrombin time, and is used to monitor warfarin levels (aim: 2.0-4.5).

IV Heparin, 5,000 units is given as a bolus then 40,000 units of heparin per 24 hours is started by infusion (continued for 3 days). 10mg oral warfarin (loading dose) is given in the evening, starting the same day (*see table*). Heparin cannot be given for longer than a few days because of the risk of throbocytopenia.

REGIME FOR ANTI-COAGULATION			
DAY 1	**DAY 2**	**DAY 3**	**DAY 4**
IV Heparin 5000 bolus 40000\24h infusion------------------------------			
Warfarin (6pm) 10mg	10mg	5mg	3mg Check INR

Check INR in the morning daily from day 4 and aim to keep it in the range of 2-3. The usual dose of warfarin needed to do this is usually in the range of 2-5mg daily. Once the warfarin dose is steady, the INR can be checked every 1-2 weeks.

Warfarin interacts with many drugs. Warfarin should not be prescribed with aspirin, which may cause gastric bleeding. The anti-coagulant effect of warfarin may be significantly increased by any of the following: dextropropoxyphene, NSAIDS, quinidine, omeprazole, tamoxifen, flutamide, ketoconazole, fluconazole, metronidazole, co-trimoxazole, chloramphenicol, ciprofloxacin, stanozolol and ifosphamide. If warfarin causes bleeding it can be reversed with vitamin K (*see Bleeding*).

IVC filter insertion may be indicated for recurrent symptomatic pulmonary emboli when anti-coagulation is contra-indicated.

DEHYDRATION

Dehydration causes:

- Reduced blood volume
- Tachycardia
- Reduced blood pressure
- Stiff skin folds\sunken eyes
- Dark urine
- Thirst (in the early stages)
- Dry mouth

Dehydration is common at the end of life, and for dying patients has some advantages:

- less urinary output
- reduced respiratory secretions
- reduced gastric secretions

However, terminal dehydration is not inevitable. In a study (in fact of hypercalcaemia) 12 out of 22 patients (not receiving IV fluids) who died within 48 hours of blood being taken, had essentially normal urea and electrolyte results (Reference: Lancet 15 September 1984 p.631).

N.B. Dying patients (day to day deterioration) rarely experience thirst or hunger. Hydration and feeding are therefore no longer priorities, and in fact can become burdensome for a very weak patient. As long as the patient is not thirsty, IV fluids are unnecessary.

Dryness of the mouth is usually the only symptom of terminal dehydration, and careful 2 hourly mouth care and ice chips to suck will solve that problem.

IV fluids have no effect on:

- life expectancy
- patient comfort
- weakness
- progress of the disease

If a patient is thirsty then re-hydration is needed, either by nasogastric tube or intravenously. Thirst is usually only a problem for patients with malignant dysphagia, who may develop dehydration when when they are still relatively active and not yet dying (week by week deterioration).

Subcutaneous fluids can occasionally have a place in management, for example if relatives insist that the patient is given systemic fluids. Subcutaneous saline can be given at 50-100ml per hour, into the anterior abdominal wall. This forms a painless lump which is soon absorbed.

Sedated patients may require IV fluids. Severely agitated patients occasionally need to be sedated for some days in the terminal phase of illness, because reducing the sedation increases the agitation and distress. In this situation, if the patient continues to survive, IV fluids may be needed, depending on the opinions of the relatives, to demonstrate that death occurs due to progression of the malignant disease and not due to dehydration.

Reference:
Regnard C, Mannix K. Reduced hydration or feeding in advanced disease – a flow diagram. Palliative Medicine 1991; 5: 161-4

DEPRESSION

Depression can be defined as low mood and low self-esteem for at least 2 weeks. It affects around 10% of hospice patients. Depression is more likely with:

- Past history of depression\alcoholism
- Family history of depression
- Poor social support
- Severe pain

Depression or appropriate sadness? Sadness requires counselling and social contact rather than medication. Low mood may be part of a normal adjustment reaction. Depression is associated with low self-esteem and inability to enjoy anything at all.

An adjustment reaction can occur after any life crisis and can cause distressing emotions (fear, anxiety, anger, misery). These feelings normally only last 1-3 weeks before the person begins to resolve them. It differs from severe depression in that the person feels bad about the situation rather than about themselves and they are able to distract themselves from their distress at times. It lasts several weeks and the patient may require counselling or psychotherapy.

Features of clinical depression, which would particularly indicate the use of an antidepressant are:

- Low self-esteem
- Lack of interest or pleasure in anything
- Expressionless face (unable to greet friends\family)
- Persistent thoughts of death\suicide
- Delusions (bizarre beliefs)

The patient may appear either withdrawn or agitated. Other features of clinical depression are less helpful because they can also be symptoms of advanced cancer: poor appetite, loss of energy, poor sleep (or excessive sleep) and poor concentration.

N.B. Depression is more likely to respond to anti-depressants plus emotional support than to emotional support alone.

Management of depression may involve:

- Support
- Counselling
- Trial of tricyclic.
- Psychiatric referral

Support is needed in times of crisis, to allow a person time and energy to find new coping strategies (*see Support*).

Counselling explores the impact of the illness on a patient's life and thinking. Referral to a psychologist or counsellor may be appropriate. Cognitive counselling approaches focus on the automatic negative thoughts that can lower mood (*see Psychological Support*). It may involve several sessions, eg 1 hour a week for 5-10 weeks. Depression is often related to the meaning of the situation for the patient. An obsessive patient may fear loss of control to the extent of withdrawing from all social interaction. A patient may be ill at the same age that their mother died. A young ill mother may feel a loss of role and purpose in life. A person consumed by guilt may only start to feel better after making a confession. Committed listening can be very healing, and can help patients to work towards doing something, either practical or symbolic, to make sense of their situation. (*see Spiritual pain*).

Tricyclics. There is little to lose from trying a tricyclic if the patient seems to be significantly depressed. Tricyclics take 5-10 days to begin to take effect. 80% experience an improvement in mood after 3 weeks. 20 % do not respond. Dose is started low, 10-25mg at night, and increased every 1-2 days up to 75-100mg at night, if the patient can tolerate the side-effects, especially the dry mouth. Protriptyline has a stimulant action. The newer tricyclics (lofepramine, dothiepin) are less likely to produce side-effects. Lofepramine is more activating and should be given during the day, 70mg daily increasing to 70mg BD or TDS. It is helpful to be familiar with a range of tricyclics.

A RANGE OF TRICYCLICS

TRICYCLIC	SEDATION
Lofepramine (Gamanil)	+
Imipramine (Tofranil)	++
Dothiepin (Prothiaden)	+++
Amitriptyline (Tryptizol)	++++

Side-effects of Tricyclics:

- Dry mouth
- Blurred vision
- Urinary retention
- Constipation
- Sweating
- Tachycardia
- Postural hypotension
- Tremor
- Confusional state

The new 5HT-uptake inhibitors, such as fluoxetine (Prozac) 20mg daily, are effective and non-sedating and have little anti-cholinergic or cardiac effects, but may cause nausea, vomiting or diarrhoea.

CLASSIFICATION OF ANTI-DEPRESSANTS

ANTI-DEPRESSANT	HALF-LIVES (hours)
Tricyclics (NA re-uptake inhibitors)	
imipramine (Tofranil)	12-24
lofepramine (Gamanil)	12-24
dothiepin (Prothiaden)	14-40
clomipramine (Anafranil)	17-36
trimipramine (Surmontil)	30-72
amitriptyline (Tryptizol)	18-96
nortriptyline (Allegron)	18-96
maprotiline (Ludiomil)	12-108
protriptyline (Concordin)	15-200
5HT re-uptake inhibitors	
fluoxetidine (Prozac)	24-140
fluvoxamine (Faverin)	13-19
trazodone (Molopaxin)	3-6
Mono-amine oxidase inhibitors	
phenelzine (Nardil)	1.5
tranylcypromine (Parnate)	2.5
Miscellaneous	
mianserin (Bolvidon)	12-29
flupenthixol (Fluanxol)	35

NA = Noradrenaline
5HT= 5 Hydoxytryptamine (sereotonin)

Psychiatric referral should be considered for severe depression with phobic features, delusions or marked withdrawal. It is best to continue inpatient care and symptom control in the hospice\palliative care unit, and for the psychia trist to visit. MAOIs can be very effective but must be used with great care and can have dangerous interactions with certain foods and drugs, including morphine. Lithium may be indicated for severe mood swings. Profound depression may be an indication for ECT.

Electro-convulsive therapy (ECT) can be very effective, especially in the elderly, and should be considered even if the prognosis is short, for depressive stupor (not eating or drinking) or delusional states. Physical frailty is not a contra-indication to treatment.

Suicide is no more common among cancer patients than the general population. Discussion of suicide is not necessarily a sign of depression, but may be a way of feeling more in control of the situation, or conveying fears.

DIABETES

Diabetes can be defined as a blood glucose above 10 mmol\l. It occurs in about 5% of patients with advanced cancer. The patient is usually a known diabetic. Other causes are:

- Steroid-induced diabetes
- Cancer of the pancreas
- Ectopic ACTH (from oat cell cancer of bronchus)

Diabetes is suspected if there is:

- Polyuria or thirst
- Drowsiness
- Increasing weakness

Oral hypoglycaemics may be enough to control mild diabetes. Sulphonylureas increase insulin secretion, provided there is some residual pancreatic function: glibenclamide (Daonil, Euglucon) 2.5-10mg daily, or in elderly patients the shorter-acting glicazide (Diamicron) 40-60mg daily. If this is insufficient, add metformin (Glucophage) 500mg TID, which increases peripheral effectiveness of insulin.

Mixtard,10 units BD, is started if diabetes remains uncontrolled, and the dose is increased according to BD measurement of glucose levels, to keep pre-prandial glucose levels below 8 mmol\l. Hypoglycaemia can still occur. Patients on insulin should be warned about symptoms or hypoglycaemia (sweating, tremor, altered behaviour) and should carry sugar.

If vomiting occurs change to soluble insulin TID, and measure capillary blood glucose (e.g. dextrostix) TID, and adjust the dose according to a sliding scale, for example:

SLIDING SCALE FOR INSULIN	
Blood Glucose (mmol\l)	Units of Insulin
10	0
10-15	10
15-20	20

Dietary restrictions can be relaxed in advanced cancer. The normal aim of dietary control is to reduce sugar intake but also to spread carbohydrate intake over the day and to cover it with insulin. Restrictions are less important when life-expectancy is short, but some longterm diabetic patients may feel psychologically better if strict control is maintained.

Weak diabetic patients who are eating little still require about 10 units of insulin BD, because the liver continues to produce glucose. Insulin can be stopped if the patient is unconscious and dying.

Reference:
Boyd K. Diabetes mellitus in hospice patients: some guidelines. Palliative Medicine 1993; 7: 163–164

DIABETES INSIPIDUS

Diabetes insipidus causes thirst and polyuria. It is a rare condition in which large volumes of dilute urine are produced due to lack of the pituitary hormone ADH (anti-diuretic hormone). It can occur, rarely, in cancers of the bronchus and breast, due to hypothalamic metastases. It can also occur in primary brain tumours. Onset can be sudden, with thirst and high volume urine output (4-10 litres a day). Diagnosis is confirmed by measuring plasma and urine osmolality and finding very dilute urine in a slightly dehydrated patient. It is treated with desmopressin.

Desmopressin (DDAVP) is synthetic ADH (anti-diuretic hormone), which acts on the renal tubules to increase water absorbtion. The dose is 300–600 micrograms orally daily (100 microgram tablets) or 1–4 micrograms by IM injection. A single dose lasts 12 hours. The strength of the dose is adjusted so that the patient produces at least 500ml of urine per day (to prevent water intoxication).

Carbamazepine (Tegretol) 100-200mg BD will also reduce urinary output in diabetes insipidus, by increasing the sensitivity of the renal tubules to circulating levels of ADH. Chlorpropamide has the same action, but doses have to be monitored carefully to avoid hypoglycaemia.

DIAMORPHINE

Diamorphine (Diacetylmorphine or Heroin) is a semi-synthetic derivative of morphine. It was first prepared in 1874, marketed in 1898 as Heroin, and banned in the USA in 1924 because of the rising number of addicts. It remains banned in most countries of the world.

Oral diamorphine is a pro-drug of morphine. It is rapidly converted to morphine in the body and is identical to morphine in its clinical effects. Studies on urinary excretion of their metabolites suggested that oral diamorphine may be slightly better absorbed than oral morphine, but this is not clinically relevant, and they are equi-analgesic. For example, a patient who is pain-controlled on 30mg oral diamorphine 4 hourly will be equivalently pain-controlled on 30mg oral morphine 4 hourly.

Diamorphine injections are used, rather than morphine injections, because of diamorphine's high solubility. 400mg diamorphine will dissolve in 1ml of water, whereas it would take 10ml of water to dissolve 400mg morphine.

The dose of diamorphine by injection is 50% of the oral dose of morphine. For example, a patient who is pain-controlled on 30mg oral morphine 4 hourly, and starts vomiting, could be given 15mg diamorphine by IM injection every 4 hours (or 90mg per 24 hour SC infusion) with exactly the same analgesic effect. Subcutaneous infusions are preferred to repeated injections (*see Subcutaneous infusions*). The table below gives the equivalent doses of oral morphine to diamorphine by injection or SC infusion over 24 hours:

EQUIVALENT DOSES OF DIAMORPHINE		
Oral Morphine or Diamorphine (4 hourly)	IM Diamorphine (4 hourly)	SC Diamorphine infusion (24 hours)
5mg	2.5mg	15mg
10mg	5mg	30mg
20mg	10mg	60mg
30mg	15mg	90mg
60mg	30mg	180mg
80mg	40mg	240mg
100mg	50mg	300mg

The indications for diamorphine injections instead of oral morphine are:

- Vomiting
- Dysphagia
- Unconsciousness

IV Diamorphine is avoided, because tolerance does develop by the IV route, for reasons that are unclear (possibly a plasma factor?) It is now well described that patients who need higher and higher doses of IV diamorphine to control pain can be transferred to a lower dose of diamorphine by the SC or oral route and pain control is restored.

DIARRHOEA

Diarrhoea means loose or watery stools. 5% of hospice patients get troublesome diarrhoea. The water content of stools only has to increase from 75% (normal) to 90% to cause severe diarrhoea. The common causes of diarrhoea are:

- Impacted faeces
- Laxative imbalance
- Abdominal malignancy

Other causes of diarrhoea are:

- Rectal tumour
- Steatorrhoea
- Recto-vaginal fistula
- Post-irradiation proctitis
- Carcinoid tumours (rare)
- Infective

Impacted faeces cause diarrhoea of small liquid faeces after a period of constipation. The treatment is disimpaction (*see Constipation*).

Laxative imbalance can cause alternating diarrhoea and constipation. If the dose of laxative has been inadequate, allowing constipation to occur, and is then suddenly increased, it causes a clearing of the hard faeces and then releases loose stools, when the patient often stops the laxative, and the cycle recurs. The treatment is a careful history and advice about laxative dosage, which needs titrating (*see laxatives*).

Abdominal malignancy can cause bowel dysfunction, with diarrhoea as well as constipation. Loperamide (Imodium), 2-4mg, 6 hourly, will normally control diarrhoea due to intra-abdominal malignancy. Loperamide is the best anti-diarrhoeal. It acts peripherally on the gut, and is more powerful than the centrally-acting opioids, such as morphine, codeine or diphenoxylate (Lomotil). An entero-colic fistula causes profuse diarrhoea, because unabsorbed small bowel contents pass straight into the colon. This can be reduced with octreotide (*see below*).

Rectal tumours cause diarrhoea consisting of discharge, blood and pus. Fybogel (or other bulking agent) can be useful to form the discharge into a soft formed stool. One sachet of Fybogel is taken in water, daily or twice daily. Rectal steroids, such as colifoam enema, BD, can also reduce the discharge (*see Steroids*).

Steatorrhoea is due to malabsorbtion of fat. Pale loose smelly motions that contain a high fat content and float. It is caused by blockage of the pancreatic duct, and occurs when enzyme secretion falls below 10% of normal. Steatorrhoea is suspected in patients with cancer of the pancreas (or occasionally other upper abdominal malignancies) with:

- No response to loperamide
- Frequent motions (4-5 per day)
- Large quantity of pale stools
- Foul-smelling
- Frothy stools that float

The diarrhoea does not respond to anti-diarrhoeal drugs but does respond to pancreatic enzyme replacement.

Pancreatic enzyme supplements contain lipase (to digest fat) protease (proteins) and amylase (carbohydrate) but it is the lipase that is important to absorb the fat. They all act in the alkaline duodenal contents and are destroyed by gastric acid, and their action is therefore enhanced by giving cimetidine 200mg, 60 minutes before meals, which can be considered if steatorrhoea is difficult to control.

PANCREATIC ENZYME PREPARATIONS		
	Lipase Units	Number needed per meal (60,000 U)
Pancrex V forte	5600	10
Creon	8000	8
Nutrizym GR	10000	6
Creon 25000	25000	2

Creon capsules (and Nutrizym GR and Pancrease capsules) contain enteric-coated microspheres which deliver a high concentration of enzyme to the duodenum, provided they are swallowed without chewing. The dose of Creon varies from 2–8 capsules per meal, depending on food intake, and is adjusted according to the frequency of bowel movements. A new preparation, Creon 2500, reduces the need for large numbers of capsules with each meal. They should be taken with food or snacks or milky drinks. Excess dosage may irritate the skin around the anus.

Pancrex V forte tablets are enteric-coated but are less effective than Creon because they tend to be retained by the stomach where they are partially inactivated by gastric acid. They also contain a lower dose of lipase than Creon.

Capsules containing pancreatin powder (Pancrex V, Cotazym) are only effective if there is no gastric acid (e.g. post-gastrectomy).

Recto-vaginal fistula causes a persistent faecal leak from the vagina. The treatment of choice is a defunctioning colostomy, but where this is not possible the leak is best managed by bowel regulation, deliberately constipating with loperamide, and then emptying the rectum with enemas (twice weekly).

Post-radiation, inflammatory diarrhoea can be settled with steroid foam enemas. Colifoam (125mg hydrocortisone per application) or Predfoam (20mg prednisolone per application) are used 1-2 times a day for 1-2 weeks.

Carcinoid tumours (rare) can cause a severe diarrhoea, due to secretion of the hormone serotonin, which does not respond to loperamide. The diarrhoea (and other features like flushing and wheezing) can be controlled with octreotide.

Octreotide (Sandostatin), 50-200 micrograms BD, by subcutaneous injection, or 300 micrograms per 24 hours by SC infusion, can control severe diarrhoea. It is a long-acting analogue of somatostatin, a hypothalamic peptide which inhibits the release of regulatory hormones and reduces gastro-intestinal secretions. Side-effects are unusual, but nausea may occur. The injections are slightly irritant, so sites should be rotated. It can be effective in other rare peptide-secreting tumours such as VIPomas and glucagonomas, and for diarrhoea due to an entero-colic fistula.

Infective diarrhoea usually occurs as an outbreak in several individuals simultaneously in a family or inpatient unit. Send stool cultures. Diarrhoea in AIDS may be due to a wide variety of infections (*see AIDS*).

Reference:
Mercadante S. Treatment of diarrhoea due to enterocolic fistula with octreotide in a terminal cancer patient. Palliative Medicine 1992; 2: 257-259.

DIET

Assessment of dietary intake is part of routine assessment. Appetite and dietary intake are rated highly when patients are asked about quality of life. Improved nutritional intake may improve mental and physical well-being.

Dietary advice is often requested and is an integral part of patient care. Referral to a dietician can be very helpful, especially if there are eating or swallowing problems. Interest in a patient's diet provides psychological support to a patient and family. An explanation of the following simple principles is often greatly appreciated:

- Encourage fluids
- Encourage fruit (fibre)
- Eat little and often
- Eat <u>when</u> hungry (a microwave helps)
- Eat whatever you enjoy (avoid boring food)
- Relax dietary restrictions (e.g. low fat diets)
- <u>Cold</u> food or drinks may be preferred.
- Strong flavours may be preferred
- Try new flavours (taste preferences change)
- No foods are harmful
- Weakness may cause embarrassment (? eat alone)

<u>Vitamin supplements</u> can help psychologically and multivitamins or high dose vitamin C, 500mg QID, for several weeks may improve the appetite.

Menu planning is important for inpatient services. Meetings of catering staff, dietetic and nursing teams to evaluate the food service can greatly improve the quality of meals in terms of presentation, temperature, palatability and choice.

Glucose supplements include <u>Maxijul</u> and <u>Fortical.</u> They are tasteless powdered glucose polymers which increase energy intake. They can be added to drinks, soups or milk puddings without changing the taste.

Nutritionally complete liquid supplements are mostly designed so that 2000ml per day will provide the normal daily requirement of protein, carbohydrate, fat, minerals and vitamins. Liquid supplements available on prescription are:

- Ensure
- Ensure Plus
- Fresubin
- Fortisip

Those available over the counter are:

- Build Up
- Complan

Supplements provide either 1 cal\ml or 1.5 cals\ml (Fortisip, Ensure Plus). They are available as 200ml cartons. They can be prescribed on an FP10 for "neoplasia related cachexia or anorexia" and prescriptions that have the letters ACBS (Approved by the Committee of Borderline Substances) added will not normally be investigated. It is best to prescribe a "variety of flavours" on the first prescription, so that the patient can discover which flavours they prefer. Flavours include:

- Fortisip (vanilla, banana, orange, tropical fruits, mushroom, neutral)
- Fresubin (vanilla, nut, peach, chocolate, meusli, mocha)
- Liquisorb (vanilla, banana, chocolate, strawberry, neutral)
- Ensure (vanilla, chocolate, coffee, eggnog, nut)

Sip feeding (50-100ml per hour) of these supplements can allow a weak patient to maintain a balanced dietary intake. Patients rarely manage more than 800ml a day. Some patients find it very helpful, other dislike the concept ("invalid food", "baby food", "prison food").

An information booklet about diet may be helpful and several booklets are available, such as "Diet and the Cancer Patient" by BACUP, 121 Charterhouse Street, London EC1M 6AA.

Alternative diets are sometimes promoted as part or a holistic approach to fighting cancer. They give the patient some control and an active way of coping. They are usually high fibre, vegetarian diets and can be difficult to manage with a colostomy or oesophageal tube. Alternative diets often include mega-vitamin, mega-mineral therapy, or herbal remedies which can be expensive. There is no evidence that these improve prognosis. Provided the diet improves morale and is not causing financial hardship or becoming a burden then it can be encouraged.

References:
Shaw C. Nutritional Aspects of Advanced Cancer. Palliative Medicine 1992; 6: 105-110.
Taylor MB *et al.* Nutritional problems and care of patients with far-advanced disease. Palliative Medicine 1989; 3: 31-38.

DRESSINGS

The ideal dressing promotes moist wound healing, by providing physical protection, warmth and moisture and encouraging gas exchange, removal of exudate and dead tissue, increased granulation and reduced risk of infection. Moist wound healing is promoted by some of the newer dressings (hydrocolloid, hydrogel, alginate, foam). Wounds cannot, and need not, be made sterile to heal.

Types of dressings include:

- Low adherence (e.g. Melolin)
- Paraffin gauze tulle
- Paraffin with chlorhexidine (e.g. Bactigras)
- Semi-permeable
- Hydrocolloid
- Hydrogel
- Alginate
- Foam
- Xerogel beads
- Activated charcoal

Semi-permeable adhesive films (Opsite, Tegaderm, Bioclusive) are transparent and waterproof, yet allow gas and vapour exchange. They are used for superficial dry wounds, and reduce soreness by acting as an artificial skin. They need to be skilfully applied to the sacral area by 2 people in order to keep the skin taught, otherwise they ruck up and can cause skin damage. There is no evidence that they speed healing.

Hydrocolloid dressings (Granuflex, Comfeel, Tegasorb, Biofilm) all differ from each other. Granuflex wafers consist of a hydrocolloid wound-contact layer, then foam, then plastic film. They reduce pain (by keeping nerve endings moist), speed healing and reduce infection. Apply with the shiny side up, leaving a 4 cm margin around the wound. Remove when bubbles of exudate start soaking through (1-7 days). The wound may appear to have enlarged at first, due to debridement, and smelly gel may be present (liquified dressing, not pus). Irrigate with warm normal saline, and apply a fresh dressing. Premature removal can damage granulations and delay healing. Granuflex paste (not on FP10) can be used to fill lightly exuding cavities. Comfeel sheets change colour when they need changing. Biofilm dressings are said to be especially absorbent.

Hydrogels (Scherisorb, Vigilon) contain a starch polymer which swells to absorb moisture. They are semi-liquid gels and need a semi-permeable dressing placed on top. Apply a thick coating of 0.5 cm. Change every 1-3 days and wash off with normal saline. They are particularly good at removing hard eschar.

Alginate dressings (Kaltostat, Sorbsan) are derived from seaweed. They absorb exudate very effectively and form a gel. Kaltostat is available as a wafer or a ribbon (rope) and it is also haemostatic and controls capillary bleeding, by releasing calcium and promoting clotting. They are useful for heavily exudating wounds, but should not be used if there is only a light exudate. The rope can be packed (loosely) into cavities.

Foam dressings. The Lyofoam sheet is useful for wounds with heavy exudate. Place smooth side down, overlapping the wound edges by 3 cm, and secure with adhesive tape. The smooth side is collapsed foam, and is very absorbent. Change the dressing when exudate is visible at the lateral edges of the dressing (after 1-5 days). Do not use on wounds with light exudate, as it will stick. Silastic foam (not on FP10) is formed by mixing a silicone base with a catalyst. The mixture is poured into a cavity and sets into a foam plug. This is an excellent method for deep cavities, to allow healing from the base of the cavity, but is expensive.

Xerogel beads (Debrisan, Iodosorb) contain a starch polymer that soaks up exudate. They are applied on a thin layer of plain gauze and covered with a secondary dressing. They can be painful to remove if the wound gets too dried out.

Charcoal dressings (Actisorb Plus, Carbonet, Lyofoam C) are claimed to reduce odour. Not on FP10.

Reference:
Drug and Therapeutic Bulletin December 1991; vol 29, No 25, pages 97-100

DROWSINESS

The causes of drowsiness are:

- Morphine
- Psychotropic drugs
- Biochemical
- Infection
- Progression of malignant disease

Morphine drowsiness is typically reversed by stimulation. Starting a conversation, the patient appears alert for a few seconds, before slowly drifting back to drowsiness. The dose of morphine should be reduced if the patient is pain-free and drowsy.

Psychotropic drugs may suddenly start to cause drowsiness even if the dose has stable for some time and has not been increased, because of worsening renal or liver function.

Biochemical causes of drowsiness include:

- Hypercalcaemia (nausea, thirst)
- Uraemia
- Hyponatraemia (*see Confusion*)

Dexamphetamine (Dexedrine), 2.5-5mg daily or BD, may rarely have a place in overcoming morphine drowsiness, when reducing the dose of morphine is not possible because of pain breakthrough. It may be especially useful if the patient wants to be alert for a particular social event. If used for longer periods there is a risk of causing side-effects of agitation, irritability, headaches and tremor.

N.B. Most patients dislike feeling drowsy. However, some patients are not distressed by it and a few even prefer drowsiness to being alert.

DYSPEPSIA

Dyspepsia (heartburn, indigestion) means epigastric or retrosternal pain, related to eating. It can be due to reflux oesophagitis, gastritis due to NSAIDs, a gastric ulcer or a duodenal ulcer.

Antacids neutralize gastric acid and can control dyspepsia due to reflux oesophagitis or gastritis. The usual dose is 10-20 ml after meals (for reflux) or between meals for gastritis. 20ml 2 hourly reduces acidity by 50% (as much as cimetidine), although it has less effect on nocturnal acidity. Liquid preparations are more effective than tablets. All are insoluble and have a slow prolonged action, except sodium bicarbonate which acts rapidly. Antacids can reduce the absorbtion of other drugs and should be given 1 hour later.

Magnesium trisilicate is slightly laxative and is therefore usually more useful than aluminium hydroxide (constipating). Large quantities can contribute to sodium retention and oedema.

Gaviscon contains an alginate which forms a layer on top of gastric contents and reduces reflux. It is ineffective with cimetidine and asilone.

Asilone contains aluminium hydroxide and dimethicone which is a antifoaming agent and reduces flatulence.

Mucaine contains a surface anaesthetic (oxethazaine) which can reduce the pain of oesophagitis due to reflux or radiation.

Ranitidine (Zantac) 150mg BD is an H2 receptor antagonist and reduces gastric acid secretion. It is useful for reflux oesophagitis and is highly effective in preventing duodenal ulceration in patients on NSAIDs, but is less effective in reducing gastric ulceration. A study of 20 healthy voluteers showed that ranitidine was most effective in preventing aspirin-induced gastric erosions if taken 2 hours before meals, and was more effective in a high dose of 600mg BD.

Ranitidine is preferred to cimetidine, which increases the effects of warfarin, phenytoin and theophylline and may be more likely to cause a reversible confusion than ranitidine. Alternative H2 antagonists such as famotidine (Pepcid PM) and nizatidine (Axid) have no advantages over ranitidine.

Omeprazole (Losec) 20-40mg daily is reserved for the 5-10% of patients who do not respond to histamine H2 antagonists. It is a proton pump inhibitor, which binds to the ATPase of the parietal cell and completely blocks acid secretion. Side-effects of headache and diarrhoea can occasionally be severe.

Misoprostol (Cytotec) 200 micrograms BD-QID can prevent NSAID-induced gastric ulceration, but does not always control the dyspepsia that can occur in 15-20% patients on NSAIDs. It is a prostaglandin analogue. It has the disadvantage of sometimes causing severe dose-related diarrhoea. It is mainly indicated for patients with a history of gastric ulceration, who are starting an NSAID.

DYSPHAGIA

Dysphagia means difficulty swallowing. It occurs in about 12% of hospice patients.

Causes of malignant dysphagia are cancers of the oesophagus, stomach or head and neck. Mediastinal nodes can cause extrinsic compression of the oesophagus. A patient with cancer can still develop a benign peptic stricture. Neurological causes of dysphagia require different management (*see Motor Neurone Disease*).

Oesophageal thrush can cause severe dysphagia, and may occur in the absense of oral thrush. It typically causes pain on swallowing hot drinks. Ketoconazole suspension 200mg daily (or BD initially) will clear oesophageal thrush in a few days, and should then be continued to prevent recurrence.

Management options for malignant dysphagia include:

- Radiotherapy
- Dilation
- Intubation,
- Laser
- Steroids
- Nasogastric feeding
- Gastrostomy

Radiotherapy (eg 30 Gy over 2 weeks) can be given to squamous cancers to reduce tumour size and improve swallowing. It can be combined with tube insertion (the tube can be inserted first) or palliative surgery to bypass the tumour (gastro-oesophageal anastomosis). Intracavity radiotherapy techniques are being developed and may be more effective.

Dilation of a malignant stricture can improve swallowing and occasionally has a place for early dysphagia (for solids) or where intubation is not possible. It takes 10-15 minutes via endoscopy. Following oesophagectomy, about 30% of patients come to need repeated dilation of the anastomosis.

Intubation improves swallowing in 90%, and should be considered in all cases of severe dysphagia. Previous radiotherapy does not preclude intubation. It can be performed endoscopically, but usually involves a G.A. and sometimes a small laparotomy to suture the lower end of the tube into place. The oesophagus has to be dilated up and there is a small risk of perforation. It is not always possible, particularly for lower oesophageal tumours, or for tumour recurrence at the site of an anastomosis following resection of the oesophagus. Patients are routinely advised to have a fizzy drink after meals. Tube problems include:

- Reflux (on lying flat)
- Blockage with food (endoscope)
- Pain (if it slips upwards) – reposition tube
- Tumour overgrowth – laser
- Disintegration (Celestin tubes)

Laser therapy can debulk tumours and improve swallowing in 90%. It may take two treatments to restore the patency of the lumen; treatment can be repeated every 4-6 weeks. Laser can be used to treat malignant overgrowth of a prosthetic tube. It cannot be used to treat dysphagia due to compression of the oesophagus by mediastinal nodes (*see Lasers*).

High dose steroids (dexamethasone 8mg or prednisolone 60mg a day) will often improve swallowing in malignant dysphagia by reducing peri-tumour oedema. Steroids may take several days to take effect. Soluble prednisolone tablets are available and dexamethasone tablets will also dissolve slowly in warm water. Dexamethasone can also be given subcutaneously (*see Subcutaneous infusions*).

Cancers of the head and neck (mouth, pharynx and larynx) can all cause dysphagia without obvious obstruction, due to extrapharyngeal infiltration and splinting of soft tissues, causing dysfunction of the swallowing reflex. Swallowing can be improved, sometimes dramatically, by high dose steroids. The mechanism may be peri-neural spread of tumour, which has been observed in post-mortem studies.

Nasogastric tube feeding can be avoided in most patients, who can usually continue to swallow a soft diet of liquidized foods or supplementary foods such as Ensure. NG feeding may be indicated if a patient is hungry or thirsty and has a patent oesophagus. This can occur due to inco-ordinate swallowing, as in some oral or pharyngeal tumours. A fine bore tube is reasonably well tolerated for a few days and does not need to be frequently changed. However, it is only indicated for short-term nutritional support. Tube displacement or discomfort occurs within 2-3 weeks in almost all patients. In one study (Park, 1992) 20 patients with dysphagia randommly allocated to have nasogastric feeding could only tolerate the tube for a median of 5 days. Oesophageal ulceration can also occur. Intermittent NG feeding for 24-48 hours every few days is another option, and can sometimes maintain hydration, without the need for other measures. Having a nasogastric tube passed is not pleasant, but this can still be the best option for some patients with a short prognosis. Discuss the options with the patient.

Percutaneous endoscopic gastrostomy (PEG) was first performed in 1980 and is a much simpler proceedure than open gastrostomy. It is performed under IV sedation and local anaesthetic. It is more acceptable to patients than nasogastric feeding and longer lasting. In one study (Park, 1992) 38 patients with a PEG ranked its acceptability as excellent (16) very good (21) or fair (1).

The technique of PEG is successful in 95% of cases, but should not be attempted if there is ascites, gastric ulcer, previous abdominal surgery or if the patient is on warfarin. Prophylactic antibiotics are given (IM cefuroxime 750mg 1 hour before the proceedure). Two operators are required. An endoscope is passed into the stomach and transilluminates the site for external skin puncture, with a cannula. A thread is then passed through the cannula and grasped by the endoscopist, and pulled up through the mouth. a fine-bore gastrostomy tube (e.g. Ponsky-Gauderer 20 Fr silicone tube, Bard International Products) is then tied to the thread and pulled back through the mouth and stomach and out through the abdominal wall. If water passes freely into the stomach, then feeding can start after 12 hours once bowel sounds are present.

Liquid food, such as Ensure, is infused slowly over several hours, by a battery-operated volumetric pump (e.g. Flexiflo, Abbott Laboratories). The infusion is started at 50ml per hour and increased to 100ml per hour by day 3. Total volume is tailored to need. Liquid feed is given by infusion to avoid the Dumping syndrome – when a sudden osmotic load in the bowel can cause hypotension and dizziness.

The tube can be aspirated every 8 hours to detect delayed gastric emptying (more than 150ml in the stomach). The main problems are wound infection, tube displacement, aspiration pneumonia and peritonitis (rare).

A tracheo-oesophageal fistula is usually a pre-terminal event. The patient tends to cough after drinking, and may cough up large quantities of fluid. An orange drink will cause orange sputum. A small early fistula can sometimes be sealed by the insertion of an oesophageal tube. Aspiration tends to cause pneumonia within a few days, when antibiotics should be normally be avoided, and any pain or dyspnoea treated symptomatically (*see Terminal phase*).

References:
Sykes NP, Baines M, Carter RL. Clinical and pathological study of dysphagia conservatively managed in patients with advanced malignant disease. Lancet September 24, 1988; page 726.
Park RHR *et al*. Randomized comparison of percutaneous endoscopic gastrostomy and nasogastric tube feeding in patients with persisting neurological dysphagia. Br Med J 1992; 304: 1406-9.

DYSPNOEA

Dyspnoea means a distressing difficulty in breathing. It is a symptom, not a sign, and can be present even if the breathing appears normal. 50% of hospice patients have dyspnoea on exertion, 75% of those with lung or pleural involvement. Severe dyspnoea (at rest) occurs in only 5%.

Dyspnoea occurs most commonly in cancers of the lung, breast, prostate, colon and rectum. In 25% of these patients there is neither lung nor pleural involvement. Mild exertional dyspnoea occurs as a feature of any advanced cancer, even with no evidence of lung disease, due to general factors such as anaemia and muscle weakness. Tumour mass, metastases, collapse, consolidation, lymphangitis or an effusion can all cause dyspnoea by reducing lung capacity or increasing lung stiffness.

The main mechanism of dyspnoea is areas of atelectasis (collapse) stimulating bronchial receptors. This causes a respiratory overdrive (which can be reduced by morphine) – *see below*.

Assessment of severity of dyspnoea is made by asking patient and relatives about limitations to normal daily activities:

- Stairs
- Walking on the flat
- Talking
- At rest?
- Panic attacks?

Examination is needed to observe the patient's breathing pattern on talking and walking and for stridor, cyanosis (blue lips and tongue) dilated neck veins, chest expansion (?symmetrical) breath sounds (?wheeze or crepitations), rib tenderness, hepatomegaly and ascites. A unilateral wheeze is a classical sign of compression of a large airway by tumour. Chest Xray and Hb level are always necessary, and ECG and lung function tests and blood gases may also be helpful. Note that normal breath sounds and a normal chest Xray can occur in anaemia, multiple pulmonary emboli and early lymphangitis, as well as in hyperventilation

Episodes of severe dyspnoea, unrelated to exertion, suggest hyperventilation but can also occur with arrythmias, pulmonary emboli and a tracheo-oesophageal fistula. Hyperventilation is very common, and is often a factor that worsens the dyspnoea. Anxiety increases the breathing rate, which worsens the dyspnoea. It is episodic and associated with feelings of panic.

Orthopnoea (shortness of breath only on lying flat) is a feature of left ventricular failure, but also occurs in ascites and bilateral diaphragmatic palsy. Most patients with dyspnoea find it is worsened on lying flat.

Reversible causes of dyspnoea must be excluded. The speed of onset can give a clue to the cause (*see table*).
Arrythmias can be initially mistaken for an episode of hyperventilation, because the patient feels dizzy, dyspnoeic and panicy. Arrhythmias can be caused by malignant infiltration of the pericardium. An ECG is necessary to diagnose the type of arrhythmia and it usually reponds to appropriate anti-arrhythmics, usually digoxin or a beta-blocker.
Pericardial effusions can occur due to malignant infiltration of the pericardium and causes dyspnoea, tachycardia, hypotension, dilated neck veins due to a raised JVP, heart sounds that are difficult to hear and an enlarged cardiac shadow on X-ray. Aspiration under ECG control in a cardiology unit may be appropriate, and subsequently a pericardial window via a median sternotomy will prevent recurrence. (Palliative Medicine 1988; 2: 62-3).

REVERSIBLE CAUSES OF DYSPNOEA

SPEED OF ONSET	MANAGEMENT
Onset over hours	
Arrythmia	ECG, verapamil digoxin or other anti-arrythmic
Heart failure	Diuretics
Bronchospasm	Bronchodilators
Pulmonary embolus	Anti-coagulation
Pneumothorax	Intercostal drain
Anxiety	Counselling
Onset over days	
Infection	Antibiotics
SVC obstruction	RT
Pleural effusion	Aspiration
Pericardial effusion	Aspiration
Tracheal compression	Stent
Onset over weeks	
Tumour growth	RT, steroids
Anaemia	Transfusion

Symptomatic treatments include:

- Radiotherapy
- Morphine
- Bronchodilators
- Steroids
- Nebulized lignocaine
- Physiotherapy
- Anxiety management
- Oxygen
- Nabilone

Radiotherapy can help if there is tumour obstructing the trachea or a main bronchus. About 40% of such patients have symptomatic improvement after RT.

Low dose morphine (2.5–20mg 4 hourly) reduces dyspnoea by an unknown mechanism. The dose can be increased 4 hourly, depending on response. CO_2 retention does not occur when morphine is used in this way. Doses above 20mg of morphine 4 hourly are unlikely to bring further benefit.

Nebulized diamorphine can sometimes reduce dyspnoea even in patients already on high dose of morphine for pain control. 5–30mg of diamorphine in 5ml saline can be given 4 hourly or used on a PRN basis. In a study of patients with COAD inhaled morphine improved exercise tolerance, and was more effective than placebo. Since only 10% of inhaled morphine is absorbed into the bloodstream, it probably acts at opioid receptors in the lung. Further studies are needed to ascertain whether inhaled morphine or diamorphine has any advantages over oral morphine for the treatment of dyspnoea (Davis C. Dyspnoea in Palliative Care. Br Med.J. 7 Nov 1992, Vol 305, p.1158.).

Slow release aminophylline such as phylocontin 225–450 mg BD may reduce the sensation of dyspnoea in addition to its bronchodilator effect, possibly by acting on the diaphragm or on cardiac output. However it is difficult to use, because there is a high risk of toxicity. Plasma levels above 110 mmol/1 commonly cause side effects (nausea, restlessness, insomnia, headache, diarrhoea, arrhythmias) and since the half-life varies from 4–25 hours, due to variable metabolism, it can sometimes cause more harm than good in terms of symptom control. Monitor carefully.

Bronchodilators are well worth trying, even if there is no obvious wheeze because there is often an element of reversible airways obstruction. In patients without bronchconstriction, there is no evidence that they reduce the sensation of dyspnoea. Consider:

- Nebulized salbutamol (Ventolin) 2.5–5mg, 4 hourly
- Nebulized ipratropium (Atrovent) 250–500 micrograms, 4 hourly

N.B. Nebulized salbutamol and ipratropium used together can precipitate acute glaucoma (pain and blurred vision) in susceptible individuals with severe hypermetropia. (Bronchodilators are discussed in more detail in the section on Cough).

Steroids in high dosage (8-16mg dexamethasone a day) can improve breathing in multiple lung metastases (by reducing peri-tumour oedema and increasing the area available for gas exchange) and in lymphangitis (when lymphatic obstruction causes stiff lungs). Steroids can also help with wheezing and SVC obstruction (*see Steroids*).

Nebulized lignocaine (5ml of 2% every 4 hours) can occasionally help (although it is more effective in controlling dry cough than dyspnoea). An ultrasound or jet nebulizer can be effective. A mouthpice should be used rather than a mask. It is most likely to help when there is diffuse lung disease affecting the alveolar J-receptors. It may help in lymphangitis. Patients should fast for 30 minutes after the treatment, to avoid aspiration, because pharyngeal numbness can occur. It is a technique that is still being evaluated and the patient should be under observation during treatment. Bupivacaine may precipitate bronchospasm in susceptible individuals.

Droplet size under 5 microns in diameter reach all parts of the lungs, down to the alveoli. It is thought that droplets need to reach the alveoli in order to reduce the sensation of dyspnoea. <u>Ultrasonic nebulizers</u> are portable and easy to use. They produce droplets between 4-10 microns. They contain a piezo-electic crystal that vibrates when a current passes through it. Placed on the surface of a liquid it sends up a mist of warmed droplets. <u>Jet nebulizers</u> produce smaller droplets, between 2-6 microns. Compressed oxygen (6L\min) draws up the liquid by the Venturi effect and disperses it into a mist of droplets. It cools the liquid, which may precipitate bronchospasm in susceptible individuals.

Physiotherapy is very important, and can reduce episodes of panic and can often extend the range of day-to-day activities. It is always helpful to teach <u>breathing exercises</u>, which focus on full expiration and lowering of the shoulders, and full inspiration which pushes the lower ribs outward and the diaphragm down and the abdomen outwards, together with relaxation techniques. This gives the patient and family a focus during episodes of dyspnoea and stops it escalating into panic. One patient said "Now when I get breathless, I know what to think". Physiotherapy can also help to <u>shift secretions</u> by percussion, vibration, coughing exercises or forced expiration. Vigourous techniques and postural drainage are not indicated as they can cause bronchospasm or short-term hypoxia.

Anxiety management is important, because dyspnoea is frightening ("Will I suffocate?") and episodes of hyperventilation can be assumed to occur at times in almost all patients with severe dyspnoea. The management of the element of anxiety is the key to controlling severe dyspnoea, and includes:

- Physiotherapy and breathing exercises
- Explanation of mechanism of dyspnoea
- Reassurance and support (repeated)
- Adapt lifestyle (occupation therapy)
- Distraction (massage, music)
- Nursing (positioning, moving)
- Environment (air movement, fan)
- Anxiolytics (lorazepam 0.5-1mg BD)

<u>Panic</u> can occur, with hyperventilation, fear of suffocation and worsening dyspnoea. Company is essential and the patient should not be left alone. An electric fan often helps pyschologically. Morphine, anxiolytics and oxygen may all be needed. Episodes of panic can be prevented or reduced by focusing on relaxation therapy and breathing exercises.

Explanation of the mechanism of dyspnoea often helps, for example: "You are noticing your breathing, rather like after running very hard, but the healthy parts of your lungs are still working well and the medication and relaxation will help to reduce the awareness of your breathing".

Oxygen will reduce dyspnoea at rest due to hypoxia. Since lung tumours, lung metastases, pleural effusion and lymphanigitis can all cause hypoxia, and since oxygen levels are not routinely measured, 100% oxygen (preferably humidified) at 5 litres\min should be given to all patients with distressing dyspnoea at rest. Nasal prongs are better than a mask which makes talking and eating difficult. Hypoxia may cause tachypnoea, cyanosis, restlessness and confusion as well as dyspnoea. Restlessness increases oxygen consumption, and therefore mild sedation may also help to ease dyspnoea. The need for oxygen can be demonstrated using pulse oximetry: Less than 90% oxygen saturation when breathing air indicates hypoxia. 95% oxygen saturation when breathing air means oxygen is unnecessary. The need for oxygen can also be assessed by a simple randomized trial. This may be worth considering if oxygen may be needed longterm and there is doubt about its effectiveness. Two staff are needed, one to randomly select either compressed air or 100% oxygen, the other to give the patient 5 minute treatments and ask the patient to record the severity of dyspnoea on a Visual Analogue Scale. (Bruera E et al, Lancet July 3 1993, Vol 342, p.13–14.)

Nabilone is a synthetic cannabinoid, used as an anti-emetic (Cesamet, 1mg capsule). It is sedative with bronchodilator properties (both anti-cholinergic and adrenergic), and in doses of 100-200 micrograms 8 hourly (specially prepared by the pharmacy) has been used to help control dyspnoea. There is a risk of arrythmias and it remains experimental.

Other drugs that have been tried to reduce the sensation of dyspnoea include benzodiazepines, indomethacin and chlorpromazine. Although there is some evidence that they may reduce the sensation of dyspnoea in healthy volunteers after exercise, studies in patients with dyspnoea have not shown any effect.

Terminal dyspnoea and panic occasionally occur despite the above measures, and require sedation. Rectal diazepam (Stesolid) 10mg or an IM injection of midazolam 5mg (or in severe panic midazolam 1mg IV) are all effective for emergency sedation. A subcutaneous infusion starting with midazolam, 20-60mg, and diamorphine 20-30mg (or more, depending on previous dose of oral morphine) per day, and increasing if necessary will effectively maintain control of distressing dyspnoea. Bubbling can occur, but usually does not distress the patient as much as the family. It can be reduced with anticholinergics (see Bubbling). A peaceful death is always possible, even though in severe dyspnoea it involves some sedation. It can be reassuring for patients to know that death can be ultimately peaceful – many fear they will suffocate to death (see Terminal phase).

The pathophysiology of dyspnoea is complicated and not fully understood. Normal breathing is maintained by rhythmic electrical activity in the respiratory centre in the brain stem, which is stimulated by mechanical receptors (stretch receptors in the bronchioles, airways, diaphragm, intercostal muscles) and by hypoxia and raised CO_2 levels in the blood (detected by chemoreceptors in the aorta and carotid).

General level of arousal affects respiratory drive – dyspnoea tends to be less severe during sleep and worse if the patient is anxious. Endogenous opioids may act as inhibitory neurotransmitters in the respiratory centre.

Hypoxia or high CO_2 both cause dyspnoea, which can be reduced by bilateral resection of the carotid bodies, which inhibits the ventilatory response to hypoxia. However, dyspnoea is not perceived, even in severe hypoxia, after C3 cord transection, which paralyses the respiratory muscles. Dyspnoea is only experienced if the lungs can respond with increased ventilation.

Respirataory muscle activity is needed for dyspnoea to occur. Exercise-induced dyspnoea in normal subjects can be reduced by local aesthetic blockade of respiratory muscles. Dyspnoea in patients can be reduced by bilateral vagal blockade (reducing input from the mechano-receptors). Inactivation of J-receptors by inhaling local anaesthetic reduces dyspnoea in chronic lung disease.

In malignant lung disease dyspnoea is usually due to distortion and stimulation of the mechanical receptors, and blood gases are often normal.

Wide variation occurs in the degree of dyspnoea experienced by both healthy volunteers (with induced breathlessness) and patients with similar degrees of of respiratory abnormality. Both anxiety and depression increase the intensity of dyspnoea. In cancer, breathlessness has a sinister significance, and therefore tends to cause much more distress than the same degree of breathlessness in a normal subject, e.g. after running up stairs.

References:
De Como F *et al.* Does pharmacological treatment affect the sensation of breathlessness in terminal cancer patients. Palliative Medicine 1991; 5: 237-243.
Ripamonti C, Bruera E. Review article. Transdermal and inhalatory route of opioid administration: the potential application in the cancer patient. Palliative Medicine 1992; 6: 98-104.

ECTOPIC HORMONES

Syndrome of inappropriate ADH (SIADH) can cause drowsiness, confusion or seizures. It occurs in about 5% of patients with small cell lung cancer and occasionally in other cancers, due to tumour peptides that mimic ADH and cause water retention and overload. The syndrome consists of:

- Hyponatraemia (serum sodium below 125mmol\l)
- Plasma osmolality less than 270 mOsm\kg
- Urine osmolality over twice that of plasma

The high urinary concentration is due to low water excretion. It is treated with water restriction (500ml per day) and demeclocycline (Ledermycin) 300mg QID, reducing to BD, which inhibits the renal tubular effect of ADH.

Ectopic ACTH is associated with small cell lung cancer, and rarely other tumours (including lung, thymus, pancreas, colon, prostate and ovary). It causes:

- Severe weakness
- Hypokalaemic alkalosis
- Elevated cortisol
- Elevated ACTH

Cortisol levels fail to suppress with dexamethasone. It is treated with metyrapone, 0.5-4g daily, which inhibits cortisol. Steroid replacement is then needed (dexamethasone 0.5-1mg daily is adequate).

Thyrotoxicosis can occur rarely due to TSH-like peptides. It has been described in choriocarcinoma, testicular, breast and lung cancers and mesothelioma.

Gastro-intestinal peptides occur in carcinoid syndrome (5HT causes wheezing, flushing and diarrhoea) and in rare secretory tumours of the pancreas, which may secrete gastrin (peptic ulceration), vasoactive intestinal peptide (severe diarrhoea, flushing) and insulin (spontaneous hypogycaemia). Octreotide can offer effective palliation for some of these symptoms (*see Diarrhoea*).

Reference:
Stein RC, Non-metastatic manifestations of malignancy: hormonal. Palliative Medicine 1989; 3: 189-196.

EMERGENCIES

Emergencies can arise in palliative and hospice and terminal care. They can cause confusion, panic and suffering for a patient and family. The management of emergency situations is therefore important, even when the treatment may not prolong life.

Psychological emergencies:

- Panic attack
- Acute confusion

Radiotherapy emergencies:

- Spinal cord compression
- Tracheal compression
- SVC compression

Medical emergencies:

- Severe pain
- Haemorrhage
- Acute dyspnoea
- Siezures
- Hypercalcaemia

Drug emergencies:

- Allergic reaction
- Dystonic reaction
- Morphine overdose

Surgical emergencies:

- Acute urinary retention
- Fractures
- Tracheal compression

Panic attacks are one of the commonest emergencies, because having cancer is frightening. Panic attacks can be terrifying and should be considered as warranting emergency management. They usually resolve in time if the patient is encouraged to express their fears, and as they adjust and mobilize resources within themselves and those around them. In the acute phase the patient may occasionally need admission if they are living alone.

Lorazepam 1mg sublingually will give a rapid anxiolytic effect, but is not a substitute for counselling and support (*see Counselling, Support*).

Acute confusion can cause severe agitation and aggression and the patient may need urgent sedation if they are in danger of hurting themselves or others, with IM 10mg Haloperidol. Terminal agitation can be resistant to medication, and a combination of diamorphine 2.5mg (or half the 4 hourly oral dose of morphine) chlorpromazine 50mg and hyoscine 0.4mg may be needed.

Radiotherapy emergencies usually need immediate high dose IV steroids (dexamethasone 30mg) and same day radiotherapy.

Severe pain is a medical emergency. The patient needs constant attention until the pain is under control. For constant pain use oral morphine or IM diamorphine for a quicker effect. If the patient is morphine-opioid naive start with 2.5mg diamorphine.

Drug emergencies may require IV hydrocortisone and IV piriton for acute allergic reactions, IV benztropine for acute dystonic reactions, or IV naloxone for severe morphine overdose (*see Morphine*).

Tracheal compression causes stridor and dyspnoea and may require treatment with a stent insertion or an emergency tracheostomy, but also may be a terminal event (*see Stridor*).

(See also Bleeding, Confusion, Spinal cord compression, SVCO, Pain, Bleeding, Dysnoea, Siezures, Hypercalcaemia and Fractures.)

Further Reading:
Oncologic Emergencies in Seminars in Oncology, Vol 16, No 6, Dec 1989, pp 461-594.

ENDOMETRIAL CANCER

Endometrial cancer causes 1000 deaths per year in the UK. It presents with abnormal vaginal bleeding (post-menopausal or inter-menstrual). The peak age is 50-70. Diagnosis is made on curettings. Treatment is by hysterectomy and BSO. 75% are cured, because it is slow-growing and presents early. Most are adenocarcinomas, the rarer tumours (sarcoma, adenosquamous) having a worse prognosis. Post-operative radiotherapy is given for poorly differentiated tumours or if there is invasion of the myometrium.

Recurrent disease commonly occurs in the vagina, as satellite nodules, (treated with vault caesium) or in the pelvic nodes, treated with external RT. Metastases to bone and lung occur late. Medroxyprogesterone, 100mg TID, will produce a 30% response rate. If that fails, combined chemotherapy can be tried (pulmonary metastases are particularly likely to respond) but has no established place in treatment.

Problems in advanced cancer of the endometrium include:

- Pelvic damage (*see Pelvic Tumours*)
- Discharge and smell
- Bleeding
- Ascites

ETHICAL ISSUES IN PALLIATIVE CARE

Ethics are the moral principles of conduct that are considered correct by a profession or group.

Medical decision-making is complex in palliative care. There is very often more that could be done for a patient to reverse organ failure, and to prolong life. Therefore setting limits to treatment is not an option in certain cases but an obligation in all cases. Where to set those limits of treatment can be difficult to define.

The role of a doctor is twofold: to restore health and to relieve suffering. When it is impossible to restore health the aims of treatment shift towards the relief of suffering.

First do no harm (primum non nocere) is the first principle of medical care. It seems obvious at first, but what is meant by "harm"? A surgeon makes an incision in order to restore health and relieve suffering, but the cut itself causes some suffering. A comparison has to be made between the harm inflicted and the good that results. This balance has to be constantly re-assessed in palliative care. Another example is family counselling which can bring short-term distress to a family, and makes them cry, but long-term brings great relief and improves their life together.

The will of the patient overrules the health of the patient. The patient is free to reject treatment. A person can write an advanced directive to state their preferences in case they become incapable of communication (*see Advanced Directives*). The patient is not free to request inappropriate treatment, such as to deliberately hasten death.

Appropriate treatment can be difficult to define. In theory it is simply a question of discussing the risks and benefits of every procedure with an informed patient. But in reality the situation can be complex. For example, a patient with an advanced pelvic cancer who develops ureteric obstruction will probably live significantly longer if a nephrostomy is performed, and may have certain symptoms controlled, such as confusion, nausea, itch or hiccup. But in living longer the patient also risks suffering in the future from advancing pelvic tumour that may cause distressing fistulas and severe pelvic pain, that can be difficult to control. The informed patient must be helped to decide on the relative benefits versus risks, but what if the patient is confused? Who will decide what is appropriate treatment? In such a case, detailed discussion is usually necessary with the patient and family and also between professional carers, in order to find the ethically correct line of action. The essential question is: "what will be of most benefit for the patient?".

Stopping treatment is ethically the same as starting treatment. Treatment is started in the hope that it will benefit the patient. If no benefit occurs, or if the benefit ceases, the treatment can be stopped. An example is the artificial ventilation sometimes given to patients with terminal motor neurone disease who develop respiratory failure. Stopping ventilation that has ceased to benefit the patient is ethical. Death is due to the underlying disease, not to the cessation of the ventilation treatment, which has become inappropriate. Allowing an inevitable death from irreversible illness to occur is different to causing death.

Futile measures should not be undertaken. For example, if radiotherapy or chemotherapy has no prospect of benefiting a patient, it should not be prescribed or condoned.

Telling the truth would seem to go without saying, yet in the past many doctors have deliberately witheld the truth, believing they were somehow protecting their patients from facts that could be so upsetting as to be harmful. However, several surveys have shown that the majority of cancer patients want to know the truth. The way the bad news is given is particularly important. Done in a brusque manner it can cause severe distress, but when opportunities are given for the patient to ask questions, and when explanation is given skilfully (*see Explanation*), the relief of knowing outweighs the distress. Discussing the truth reduces fear and uncertainty (the hardest emotion to bear), avoids deceit (which damages family relationships) and allows the person to attend to unfinished emotional business, to put their affairs in order and to plan for death.

Reference:
Gilhooly M *et al.* Truth telling with dying cancer patients. Palliative Medicine 1988; 2: 64-71.

Quality of life can be defined as a comparison of hopes versus experience, or as a description of a person's present lifestyle when compared to their ideal lifestyle ("What would you be doing today if you were well?"). Quality of life is different to meaning of life. A poor quality of life does not make a person's life meaningless or worthless. Quality of life is subjective, and cannot be assessed by observation. Simple measurements of physical independence do not equate with quality of life. Patients who are profoundly handicapped may still have a feeling of well-being and may rate their quality of life as high.

A simple global assessment of all aspects of quality of life cannot be made, because it is a concept that is specific to an individual and it changes with time and circumstances. Quality of life is not a useful concept when formulating policies, except a policy to make patient care as flexible as possible. But a simple question (e.g. "How would you rate your quality of life today?") can be useful when assessing the results of trials, e.g. comparing the effects of different chemotherapy treatments. Simple assessments of selected aspects of quality of life are also important when giving advice about risks versus benefits of a particular treatment, and should be routinely enquired about when discussing treatment options with a patient.

Questionnaires about quality of life (see Assessment of the patient) are more useful when attempting to relieve distress, and may themselves improve a patient's quality of life by focusing on the patient's priorities, which may relate to activity, daily living, physical health, support or outlook. The most significant questions seem to be those relating to mood and spirits. Patients tend to score their quality of life higher than observing doctors or nurses, probably because patients have lower expectations.

Quantity of life may be more important than quality of life. Some patients, even with advances Illness, want to pursue agressive treatments with little chance of benefit and sometimes with unpleasant side-effects. If this is the patient's informed choice it should be respected

References:
Fowlie M et al Quality of life in advanced cancer: the benefit of asking the patient. Palliative Medicine 1989; 3: 55-59.
Twycross RG. Quality before quantity – a note of caution. Palliative Medicine 1987; 1: 65-72.

Voluntary euthanasia means the direct intentional killing of a patient at his or her request. It remains illegal throughout the world, although it is being increasingly tolerated in the Netherlands. Such a medically assisted death is claimed to be the solution for individuals who can no longer tolerate an existence of illness. It is advocated by some as a way of increasing a person's right to self-determination. However, an individuals right to be killed would impose an unacceptable duty, presumably on doctors, to kill. Killing would become a therapeutic option. This would be open to abuse, and would put considerable pressure on those who felt a burden. It would increase the rights of a very small minority at the expense of the majority, who would be pressurized into questioning their right to future care. For many a "right to die" would become a "duty to die". Patient's who say "let me die" are generally in fear of inappropriate life-prolonging treatments rather than wanting to be actively killed. Where palliative care and symptom control and psychological support has been made available, legalized euthanasia would be a negative solution to a problem that can be solved by appropriate care.

Reference:
Saunders C. Editorial: Voluntary euthanasia. Palliative Medicine 1992; 6: 1-5.

Research is ethical if studies are well designed. For example, in a comparison of two treatments, both should benefit the patient in some way. It is important that trials are randomized, as far as possible. Patients with advanced illness are often particularly keen to help with research projects, and there are many important questions that remain unanswered. However, in the hospice setting many patients will die before research projects are completed, so multi-centre studies are important to achieve statistically significant results.

The cost of care means financial choices have to be made. There is a finite amount of money available. Therefore decisions have to be made about the relative importance of care for different groups of patients. Who should take preference? Should kidney transplants take preference over special care baby units, for example? It is for society to make such decisions after prolonged and informed public debate. The duty of clinical doctors should remain primarily to provide the best available care to their individual patients. It is also a doctor's ethical duty to use the most economical and efficacious treatment available.

EXPLANATION

Explanation is an essential part of symptom control. Before about 1930 the main role of a doctor was explanation of disease processes, and the support of the sick patient. Explanation involves teaching, and the following hints may be helpful:

Ask questions first – find out what the patient already knows and what the patient wants to know.

Be simple – a patient can rarely remember more than 2 pieces of new information. Use categories e.g. "There are 2 things I want to tell you. First...."

Avoid jargon – assume that the patient may not understand your words, especially medical words.

Repeat important information – and ask the patient to repeat, to check their understanding.

Use diagrams – and give them to the patient to keep. If a thing is "in hand" it feels more in control.

Be available for further discussion or explanation to relatives.

Information leaflets can significantly improve a patient's knowledge and understanding. (Reference: Walker JR. A study to develop and assess the value of a leaflet on pain control for cancer patients taking MST in the community. Palliative Medicine 1992; 6: 65-73.)

Explaining bad news means changing someone's future for the worse. It has to be done in a balanced way. Unrealistic reassurance destroys future trust, but on the other hand, giving too much information too soon can cause anxiety and anger. The principles are:

- Arrange privacy and sit down
- Arrange for family member to be present
- Ask questions first
- Explain, using kind words
- Answer questions
- Offer future availability
- Enquire about future emotional support

Explaining bad news paradoxically often brings relief, because uncertainty is the hardest of all emotions to bear. Many patients make comments like "It was easier once we all knew what was wrong". However, adjusting to bad news takes several weeks or months.

The way bad news is given can upset patients and families for months. Giving some time is one way to demonstrate empathy. In a postal survey of 800 patients in 1991 by CRMF, 24% of patients were told the life-changing news about their diagnosis of cancer in a brief conversation that lasted less than 5 minutes. Explaining bad news brings a responsibility to offer support.

EYE PROBLEMS

Dryness of the eyes and even corneal ulceration can occur if the eyelids are unable to close properly. Use hypromellose eyedrops (artificial tears).

Blurred vision may be due to:

- drugs
- cataract
- choriodal metastasis

Blurred vision may simply require a new prescription for reading glasses. Steroids can alter the refraction of the lens. It may be due to excessive anti-cholinergic drugs (tricyclics, phenothiazines, atropine, hyoscine). Cataracts may be worsened by steroids, over a period of months. If a patient is awaiting a cataract extraction and lens implant this can be easily and quickly performed under local anaesthetic and may be well worthwhile even if the patient has a short prognosis. Choroidal metastases can cause blurred vision and respond to RT.

Double vision (diplopia) due to cranial nerve lesions sometimes occurs with bone secondaries in the base of the skull (seen most commonly in breast cancer) and may respond to radiotherapy or high dose steroids. Rarer causes are raised ICP (causing pressure on the sixth nerve) and malignant infiltration of the meninges (*see Meningeal metastases*).

Field defects (hemianopia), with loss of peripheral vision to one side, (either left or right) commonly occurs in brain tumours. The patient tends to bump into things on the affected side, and may fear blindness. Central vision is not lost.

Eye pain suggests a retro-orbital metastasis. There may be proptosis (protrusion of the eyeball). The diagnosis is made by CT scan. Early radiotherapy can prevent blindness.

Radiotherapy to the orbit does not affect vision, as the eye is radio-resistant, apart from the lens which must be shielded during treatment to prevent cataract formation.

FAMILY SUPPORT

A family can be defined as an emotionally inter-dependent group of people with a shared history, commonly held beliefs, a life-cycle of development and a future together. There are many different types of family structure, and it can be helpful to ask "Who else belongs to your family?".

A family is an inter-related system and changes to one individual affect all the family. In a crisis a family tends to use familiar methods of coping and resists change, which feels threatening. Terminal illness and death inevitably cause changes and so a period of stressful instability follows. A new pattern of family behaviour must be discovered and adopted. Initially this new behaviour may be either adaptive or dysfunctional.

Dysfunctional behaviour within a family is an attempt to protect individuals from the effects of the change, but instead it causes further disturbance and change. Eventually the family comes to find a new pattern of stability, but sometimes needs outside help to do so.

Family-centred care is essential. Illness affects all the family and therefore care is most effective when it is family-centred. Patients often feel isolated by their illness and cut off from their normal roles and relationships. Helping families to communicate can reduce feelings of isolation. Concern for the family is directly supportive to most patients, whose main concern is usually their family. Most patients want to be understood (and understand themselves) in the context of their families. Also, many relatives have so many worries that they are in effect patients as well (often attending their GP for symptoms of anxiety).

A family tree (genogram) serves several useful functions. It demonstrates interest in a person, emphasizes that the family is the unit of care and records useful family information in the notes for all the professional team. Important information frequently comes to light, such as:

- Support available
- Insight of family members
- Children's insight
- Previous deaths in the family
- Other family worries
- Unfinished emotional business
- Expectations (e.g. new grandchild)

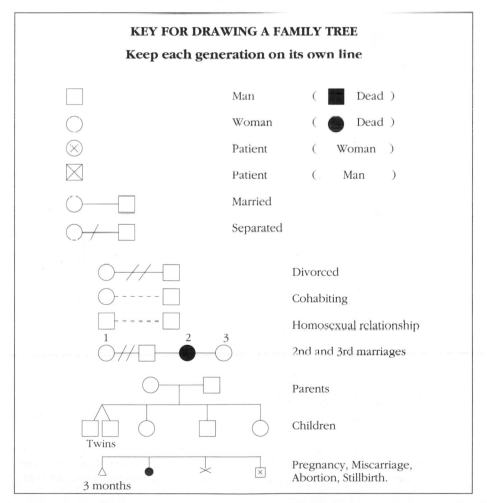

KEY FOR DRAWING A FAMILY TREE

Keep each generation on its own line

☐ Man	(■ Dead)	
◯ Woman	(● Dead)	
⊗ Patient	(Woman)	
⊠ Patient	(Man)	
◯—☐ Married		
◯⁄—☐ Separated		

Divorced

Cohabiting

Homosexual relationship

2nd and 3rd marriages

Parents

Children

Twins

Pregnancy, Miscarriage, Abortion, Stillbirth.

3 months

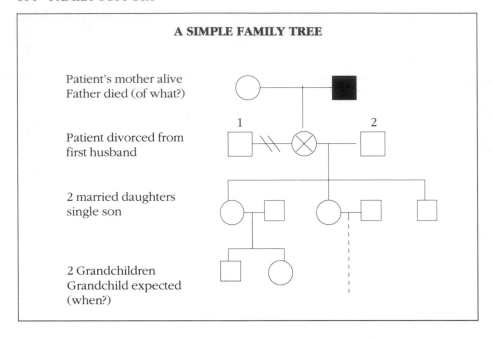

A SIMPLE FAMILY TREE

Patient's mother alive
Father died (of what?)

Patient divorced from
first husband

2 married daughters
single son

2 Grandchildren
Grandchild expected
(when?)

A family conference convened during a crisis will reduce family anxieties, (which are often about poor communication and fears of upsetting each other. A meeting usually allows a family to solve its own problems. Families that are brought together will talk together. A family conference helps the family adjust by:

- Sharing feelings
- Focusing on strengths and resources
- Gathering information

A specific invitation is needed: "We would like to meet you and any of your family you would like to have with you". Even if the offer is not accepted, it is a significant message about the focus of concern.

Families need information. One study recorded questions at 50 consecutive family conferences, and showed that most families wanted information about life expectancy (84%), extent of the illness (72%), possible future complications (50%) and many other areas (see Table).

The impact of terminal illness on a family is profound. Concern for the whole family is a very effective form of preventive health care, because unresolved bereavement adversely affects both future mental and physical health. Many families initially doubt their ability to cope at all. Balance is disturbed as the family imagines a future without one person. New ways of coping have to be considered and some families have fearsome arguments.

Family arguments need to be seen positively – they are a sign that a family is attempting to solve its problems. The crisis of terminal illness often comes

INFORMATION COMMONLY REQUESTED AT A FAMILY CONFERENCE

- Life expectancy
- Extent of illness
- Confimation of diagnosis
- Curable if detected earlier
- Possible future events
- Treatment options
- Home nursing help
- Pain
- Medications
- Can family manage at home
- Chances of recovery
- Diagnosis
- Patient's emotions
- Reasons for decline
- Radiotherapy
- Possible discharge date
- How to handle death at home
- Nutritional support
- Medical follow-up
- Equipment at home
- Bowel problems
- Other symptoms
- What to do in emergency
- Talking with children
- Communication with family members
- Financial or legal worries
- Making a will
- When death will occur
- How death will occur
- Funeral arrangements
- Genetics

Reference:
Miller RD, Krech R, Walsh TD. The role of a palliative care service family conference in the management of the patient with advanced cancer. Palliative Medicine 1991; 5: 34-39.

on top of other major events in the life-cycle of the family (childbirth, adolescents leaving home, dependent elderly parents, other illness or deaths) and we need to ask "What else is happening in your life together as a family at the moment?".

Stress in a family prevents decision-making, reduces communication, and alters roles and reactions to each other. The emotional distance between a couple can change because of illness, and for some there is an almost violent re-assessment of the marriage relationship once the future hope that "it may all be better one day" is lost. Some families initially refuse to contemplate death, feeling it is disloyal not to go on hoping. But it is possible to plan for the worst as well as to go on hoping for the best, and to discuss rather than ignore problems (*see Grief*).

Communication problems in families are common, and produce such comments as:

- Please don't tell him, he'd never cope
- It would only upset her
- She doesn't care
- He's behaving very badly
- We don't know what to say
- Talking won't change anything
- He mustn't see me cry
- We don't have morbid talk in this family

Openness about feelings becomes more difficult for all families in a prolonged crisis because of emotional exhaustion (dealing with many new situations and problems) and because of fears about upsetting oneself and others. It is very tempting for professionals to collude with a family's avoidance, but distress is inevitable and worse when it is carried alone rather than shared. Family counselling is needed if communications problems are causing distress to individual family members.

Family counselling sometimes involves being cruel in order to be kind. Emotional distress has to be exposed before it can be resolved by a family. Unresolved emotional conflict around the time of a death can cause psychological disturbances for years. Trying to somehow control emotional pain as if it were physical pain is both impossible and demoralizing for staff.

Inappropriate behaviour in a family often relates to previous experiences of loss, when insufficiently resolved mourning is re-awoken by the present distress. Such losses need to be discussed, but they are painful, so the family deviates away from them and manipulates the conversation back to safer areas like the present problems in the family. But if the family's coping strategies are not working they need to be gently challenged if they are to find new ways of coping.

Challenging does not mean disagreeing, it means asking questions that no-one has dared to ask before. The way forward is to make it safe enough to share painful memories. This involves forming a trusting relationship with the family (which is not necessarily time-consuming), and then repeatedly affirming the family before challenging them. The therapist has to convey empathy, and the conviction that the issue of change is very important and worth some distress. The style of challenging may involve comments like:

- Who is close to who in your family?
- Who is good at getting their own way?
- Who would be most upset if X were not being angry?
- What might change if Granny could appear?
- Why do you always rescue X, by interrupting?
- If you had to part, what would you regret not saying?

Family therapy techniques that may be used to promote change can include:

- Drawing a family tree
- Role play
- Sculpting
- Empty chair techniques
- Moving positions within the room

When emotional problems are tackled in this way it is best to have 2 therapists working together. Sessions of an hour per week for 2 or 3 weeks may be sufficient.

A parent with terminal illness may need advice from a social worker about childminders, playgroups, nurserys, adoption, fostering, help in the home and future care of the children. Knowledge of children's legislation can be invaluable. An experienced counsellor can also work with the children and parents at the right stage to prepare them for the loss.

Children have special needs. Their concepts of death are age-related. Young children (under 3-5 years) see death as desertion, older children search for causes and may imagine that death occurs because of something they said or did ("magic thinking"). Children express their feelings, solve problems and develop through play. They think in practical terms, not in terms of concepts. Children cope well with loss if they have access to all the information they need to adjust, and are included in the family's experience, and should be included in all family discussions. They are confused by secrecy and being excluded, which often happens both to protect the children, and also to protect adult family members from witnessing the distress of the children.

Bereaved children are at serious risk of psychological disorders (Br J Psychiat 1985; 147: 188-94). Those most at risk are in the 3-5 age group and adolescents. The impact of loss depends on the strength of attachment, which may be as strong to a grand parent as to a parent. Anger may get acted out (e.g. naughtiness at school) if the child is not encouraged to grieve by asking questions and expressing feelings. Children who are included at the time of the death can provide a lot of support to others whereas children who are denied the opportunity to be supportive often regret it later. Children of all ages should attend the funeral.

Talking with young children has to happen through the parents, who must not be displaced by the counsellor. Encouraging young children to communicate may involve using drawings, toys or puppets ("Mummy went away like this, because..."). Children imitate, and therefore respond to a counsellor willing to tell stories and chatter freely. It can reduce fears for young children (and introduce some fun) if the counsellor makes deliberate mistakes and allow the child to correct them. Ask "What happens when?" (not "How did you feel when?"). Dilute small doses of serious things with some fun. Children usually have their own bizarre fantasies about why death has occured or what it means for the future. These need to be explored and corrected. Explanation needs to be in simple direct language (e.g. "When he dies he will stop moving and breathing") and may require analogies ("It's a bit like..."). Colouring books can be useful for young children, with topics like:

- Here is our family
- Here is ... who is ill
- Here are my friends
- Here are some of the people looking after ....
- Have you noticed anything different about ....
- Things I can do to help.

Such books can be a focus for discussions about what has changed, what has not changed, what supports will remain for the future and about feelings. Children with cancer have special needs which have been reviewed in detail elsewhere (J Child Psychol Psychiat 1986; 27: 145-180).

Sitting at the death bed of a loved person is a profound and intense emotional experience. Events around this time have a bigger impact than normal and memories of these events are usually powerful and long-lasting. It is an opportunity for a family that is divided to come together again, and can be a healing opportunity for them, but this usually requires some professional guidance, without which family rifts can worsen in the emotionally charged atmosphere around the time of a family death.

After a death a family usually needs support and many need (but dare not ask for) time to be with the dead person (sometimes several hours) and time to ask questions about what has happened and what happens next. This family support is often missing, especially in busy hospital wards, but makes a considerable difference to a family.

Further Reading:
Jenkins H. The family and loss: a systems framework. Palliative Medicine 1989; 3: 97-104.
Earnshaw-Smith E. We don't need to be God after all. Palliative Medicine 1987; 1: 154-162.
Smith N. the impact of terminal illness on a family. Palliative Medicine 1990; 4: 127-135.
Cooklin AI. Tenderness and toughness in the face of distress. Palliative Medicine 1989; 3: 89-95.
Kirschling JM ed. Family based palliative care. 1990. New York. Howarth Press. 109 pages.
Ackworth A, Bruggen P. Family therapy when one member is on the death bed. Journal of Family Therapy 1985; 7: 379-385.

FINANCES – A CHECKLIST

Financial problems are important. Few patients have all their financial affairs in order when they become ill. Financial worries may be severe and complex. This checklist emphasises the need for expert advice from an experienced social worker. I am grateful to Tess Kennedy CQSW for help with this section.

The main benefits are:

- Disability Living Allowance
- Attendance Allowance

Form DS1500 (completed by a doctor), allows patients with a terminal illness (i.e. suffering from a progressive disease and not expected to live longer than 6 months) to get these benefits immediately, even if they do not yet need help looking after themselves. The doctor is asked to provide information, not a prognosis. Another doctor decides if the patient qualifies under the special rules.

Basic Income, that is not means-tested, include:

- Sickness Benefit (from DSS for 28 weeks)
- Statutory Sick Pay (from employer for 28 weeks)
- Invalidity benefit (after 28 weeks sickness)
- Severe Disablement Allowance
- Pension
- Widows Benefit

Disability benefits include:

- Invalid care allowance (paid to carer if attendance allowance has been awarded)
- Industrial injury benefit
- Child benefit
- Community Charge exemption (if mentally incapacitated)
- Christmas bonus
- Charitable grants

Other financial considerations include:

- Contract of Employment
- Medical retirement
- Pension advice
- Mortgage payment support
- Insurance policies and claims
- Arrears, debts
- Maintainance orders

Means-tested Benefits include:

- Income support
- Housing Benefit
- Family Credit
- Free prescriptions\fares\dental\optical treatment
- Funeral payment

Industrial compensation is most commonly an issue in mesothelioma and can be complicated. A civil claim can be made for compensation from the employers if:

1. The company is still trading and insured, and
2. Legislation was in force against the use of asbestos at the time the patient worked there.

It is essential to employ a solicitor who is experienced in these types of claims, and advice should be sought from The Society For The Prevention of Asbestosis and Industrial Diseases (SPAID), 38 Draper's Road, Enfield, Middlesex EN2 8LU. Telephone 0707 873025.

If the company is no longer trading it may still be possible to get an award from the department of Employment. Industrial benefit should be claimed as soon as possible from the DSS. If Industrial benefit is refused it is possible to appeal, and a specialist solicitor may still be able to obtain some compensation from employers.

A full signed statement should be made by the patient as soon as possible, detailing his work and contact with asbestos, precautions at the time, witnesses etc. A post-mortem has to be ordered by the coroner.

Making a will can help a person prepare for death and can enable a family to discuss what is happening. Families are frequently frightened to discuss the will "in case it upsets him" and yet the patient is usually very relieved when finally helped to discuss it and to leave their financial affairs in order. Even a simple makes it much easier to settle the deceased's affairs. A will is an important document, which may be challenged later, and there are complex rules regarding the signing, and a solicitor should therefore be involved.

The person must have "testamentary capacity", i.e. have a full understanding of his or her assets and be able to identify family members. If the patient is confused at times, a will made in a "lucid interval" is still legal. Many confused patients are confused later in the day but less confused or completely alert in the mornings. Any valid will signed in the presence of two witnesses cancels all previous wills. Marriage cancels all previous wills.

If the patient is unable to write, then any definite mark on the paper is acceptable, provided two witnesses add certain words, as advised by the solicitor.

The executor of the will has the task of gathering assets, paying off any debts and fees and distributing legacies. The solicitor commonly acts as executor. Money can be released from accounts either by showing the death certificate obtained from the registrar (for small amounts), or a Grant of Probate from the Probate Registry in London.

Further reading:
Ennals S. 1991: Understanding Benefits. London: British Medical Journal.

FISTULAS

A fistula is an abnormal connection between a hollow organ and the surface of the body, or between two hollow organs. It may be due to malignancy or follow RT or surgery.

Bypass surgery should be considered whenever possible for the distressing symptoms of malignant fistulas. A colostomy or a urinary diversion may be possible.

A colostomy bag can be placed over a fistula with a heavy discharge, in order to collect the fluid.

Smell may be reduced by metronidazole or other measures (*see Smell*).

Barrier creams are helpful to reduce skin soreness.

Facial fistulas can sometimes be plugged with a moulded occlusive dressing. Refer to the orthodontist.

FRACTURES

Pathological fractures occur at the site of bone metastases, most commonly in cancers of the breast, bronchus, prostate and kidney. Fractures may occur with no preceding pain.

Diagnosis is based on a history of sudden pain and\or deformity, with bony crepitus on examination, and is confirmed by Xray.

Management options include:
- Internal fixation (surgical)
- External stabilization (plaster, splints)
- Skin traction
- Local injection

Internal fixation is the treatment of choice. Methods include hip prosthesis, pin and plate or intramedullary nail and depend on the site of the fracture. Curettage of affected bone and replacement with methyl methacrylate cement may also be necessary. Surgical stabilization is not possible for pelvic fractures which are treated with RT to reduce pain and increase the chance of healing. Surgical stabilization of the spine is more difficult and less effective than for long bones, but anterior or posterior vertebral decompression may both be indicated (*see Spinal Cord Compression*). Prophylactic fixation is indicated for femoral metastases since surgery is technically easier before the bone has fractured. The presence of metal or cement does not interfere with subsequent RT.

Healing of pathological fractures is slower than normal but occurs in 50% of cases following fixation and RT, especially in breast metastases. Pain relief occurs after fixation, even in the absence of healing.

External stabilization using splints, slings or plaster of Paris may be needed if surgical fixation is not possible. High fractures of the humerus may need to be stabilized externally and a lightweight plastic support that is removable, with velcro fasteners, is then very useful. Heavy plaster splints or complex splinting such as a Thomas's splint for fractures of the femur are not usually appropriate in terminal illness.

Skin traction can be useful to manage a fractured femur in a bedbound patient, to reduce pain on movement. A 5–10kg weight (eg a catheter bag filled with water) is adequate. Diazepam or midazolam may be helpful to reduce muscle spasm around the fracture.

Local injection of 10ml 0.5% bupivacaine and 80mg (2ml) methylprednisolone (Depomedrone) into the periosteum at the fracture site can reduce pain on movement, and is worth considering if the fracture is painful despite skin traction.

Rib fractures are best treated with a single shot of 10 Gy external radiotherapy, or a local intercostal nerve block (*see Nerve blocks*).

Pelvic fractures, such as through the pubic ramus cannot be immobilized but RT, such as 25 Gy in 5 fractions, can reduce pain and speed healing.

Vertebral collapse, even if painless, is worth irradiating in order to prevent further collapse and cord compression. RT is of no benefit for established cord compression due to vertebral collapse, which requires surgical stabilization (*see Spinal Cord Compression*).

Reference:
Chalmers D. The management of bone metastases: orthopaedic procedures. Palliative Medicine 1987; 1: 121-127.

GLIOMAS

Gliomas are primary brain tumours. They arise from the supporting glial cells in the brain (not the neurones). Astrocytomas are by far the commonest gliomas in adults. They cause about 3000 deaths per year in the UK. The peak age is 50-60. The prognosis is worse in the elderly. Presentation may be with:

- Neurological loss
- Seizures
- Headaches and vomiting (raised ICP).

Diagnosis is by CT scan. Biopsy is important to grade the tumour (but may not be possible with deep-seated tumours). 80% are rapidly growing (grade 3 and 4), 20% are slow growing (grade 1 and 2).

Rapidly growing tumours (grade 3 and 4) generally cause death within 6-12 months whatever treatment is given, and only 10% survive 1 year. Surgery aims to relieve symptoms of raised ICP, either by de-bulking the tumour or by the insertion of a ventriculo-peritoneal shunt. Repeat de-bulking may be possible if the tumour is in a "silent" area (non-dominant temporal or parietal lobes). Radiotherapy can be given as a short course, 3000cGy in 10 fractions (since prognosis is too short for late side-effects to be a problem). Patients under 50 who have a complete resection followed by RT, with minimal neurological deficit have a 3 year survival rate of 20%. Severe disability (irreversible neurone damage) or age over 60 are usually contra-indications to treatment. Chemotherapy is of little value. Lomustine (CCNU) can produce a response in a small number.

Slow growing tumours (grade 1 and 2) have a better prognosis. Radiotherapy prolongs survival. Following treatment with radiotherapy 50% survive 5 years, 20% 10 years. 6000cGy over 6 weeks avoids the late side-effects of brain irradiation (dementia). Radiotherapy treatments require wide margins because the tumours infiltrate diffusely. Early disease and slow-growing oligodendrogliomas may be curable.

Deterioration is usually due to the progress of the disease but may be due to a blocked shunt, post-ictal paralysis or the wrong steroid dose.

Metastases do not occur outside the CNS, with the rare exception that patients with a shunt can sometimes develop bone metastases. Patients with proven primary brain tumours can donate kidneys for transplant (*see Organ donation*).

Advanced brain tumours cause a steady decline in function, a blunting of emotions and intellect and increasing dependency. Personality change is often the hardest part for the relatives. Particular problems in advanced disease are:

- Paralysis\speech problems
- Urinary incontinence
- Seizures
- Hemianopia
- Headaches
- Steroid side-effects

GRIEF

Grief is a normal pyschological response to any emotionally significant loss. The effects of grief are now well recognized and described briefly below. The effects do not occur as neat "stages" but tend to recur and overlap unpredictably, and need to be worked through, and worked at. Grief is one of the most intensely painful human experiences. Grief work consists of:

- Overcoming numbness
- Experiencing the emotional pain
- Learning new skills
- Re-investing emotional energy

Numbness (lack of emotional response) is often experienced, especially after a sudden loss. It may last days or weeks. This denial phase can be overcome by talking about all the events around the time of the loss. This allows the person to begin to experience their emotions.

Anxiety and restlessness occur, similar to the searching behaviour seen in animals separated from their mother. This can occur in episodes for some weeks, occasionally months. The person is distracted and unable to concentrate. A wide range of symptoms can occur including insomnia, forgetfulness, poor appetite, palpitations, breathlessness, tightness in the chest and often hallucinations of the dead person (in 50%). It is often reassuring to a grieving person to know that these are normal reactions, and that they are not going mad.

Adjustment to a different world has to occur, both practically and emotionally and takes months to years. New practical problems arise and need to be solved in new ways with new skills, and this learning process takes time (but can, in the end, be rewarding as well as frustrating). Emotional adjustment involves facing and working through strong feelings such as rejection, anger, guilt ("If only...") or loneliness.

Re-investment of the emotional energy signals the healthy end of the grief process, and may takes 2-3 years after a major bereavement. The individual can begin to think of the dead person without so much pain, and form new attachments without guilt.

Dying also involves grieving. As patients face increasing weakness and dependency, it is helpful to apply this model of grieving to their psychological distress. To quote Colin Murray Parkes: "Dying involves the gradual adjusting to a whole series of losses and disappointments. Each loss causes grief. Very often the earlier losses are harder to cope with than dying itself". Small losses, as well as large ones, cause a similar process of numbness (denial), emotional distress and then a period of adjustment.

Anticipatory grief work is important. Sudden deaths cause a more profound bereavement reaction because there is less time to adjust (Br J Psychiat 1985; 145: 424-8). But terminal illness offers time. The patient and the family are both grieving for a lost future. Sharing their sadness together reduces the patient's isolation and provides healing memories for the family. Some families are very frightened that such a conversation could somehow be damaging. But skilful counselling, which allows a family to feel in control about how much information is discussed, can bring a family closer together and allow them to support each other (*see Family Support*).

There is no "correct" reaction to a loss, which depends upon the emotional significance of the loss, the personality of the person, previous life experiences (especially of other losses), concurrent life stresses and the support available. Most importantly a person needs time and space to adjust to the loss in their own way (*see Support*).

Further Reading:
Worden JW. Grief Counselling and Grief Therapy. 1982 London: Tavistock.

HALLUCINATIONS

Hallucinations are illusions of perceptions in the absense of sensory input. To elicit whether a patient is experiencing hallucinations, a useful question is "Have you seen or heard anything strange recently?"

The causes of hallucinations are:

- Morphine
- Confusion
- Schizophrenia

Morphine in too high a dosage usually causes drowsiness, but occasionally causes nausea and can rarely cause mild hallucinations (usually visual) before drowsiness occurs. The rule in a patient on morphine is "if the patient is painfree and drowsy, or hallucinating - reduce the dose".

Confusion can cause misperceptions (eg a tie is mistaken for a snake) and this can appear as though the patient is hallucinating (*see Confusion*).

Schizophrenia typically causes auditory hallucinations (voices), delusions (bizarre beliefs) and paranoia. The patient will usually be a known case of schizophrenia on medication. Terminal agitation in such patients can require massive doses of sedatives (*see Terminal agitation*).

HEAD AND NECK CANCERS

Head and Neck Cancers include cancers of the larynx, pharynx, mouth, salivary glands, nasal sinuses and orbit. Most are squamous. They are more common in smokers. Most are treated initially with radiotherapy, except early oral cancers, which can be treated surgically. The overall cure rate is about 40%.

Recurrent tumour can develop more than 5 years after apparent cure. Recurrence in cervical nodes is treated by block dissection, which is usually a palliative procedure (to reduce pain and disfigurement) but is occasionally curative. After block dissection recurrence occurs in 25%, which may occur in other nodes or as distant metastases, especially to the lung.

Chemotherapy can be useful for local recurrence after surgery or RT. The standard drug combinations include cisplatin, bleomycin, fluorouracil and methotrexate. Reponse rates vary from 20-40%, lasting about 3 months. Response is monitored by clinical measurement, and Chest Xray if lung metastases are present.

Problems in advanced cancers of the head and neck include:

- Disfigurement
- Pain
- Bleeding
- Dysphagia
- Base of skull involvement
- Facial fistula
- Infection
- Tracheal obstruction

Dysphagia can occur without pharyngeal obstruction due to nerve involvement and splinting of the pharynx wall. It can respond to high dose steroids (*see Steroids*).

Base of skull involvement occurs most commonly with nasopharyngeal cancers and can cause cranial nerve lesions (double vision, dysarthria). It can be treated with radiotherapy.

Facial fistulas can sometimes be plugged with a moulded occlusive dressing. Ask the local orthodontist.

Infection can cause smell (*see Smell*) or pain. A throbbing pain that is not responding to morphine can be due to a bacterial infection and responds to a broad-spectrum antibiotic. The WBC may not be elevated. (Reference: Bruera E. Intractable pain in patients with advanced head and neck tumours: a possible role of local infection. Cancer Treat Rep 1986; 70: 691-2).

Tracheal obstruction causes increasing stridor and eventually hypoxia. Treatment options include steroids, radiotherapy, laser, stent or tracheostomy (*see Stridor*), but it may be a terminal event best managed symptomatically.

HEPATOMA

Hepatoma is a primary cancer of the liver. It causes about 500 deaths per year in the UK (and about 1 million deaths per year worldwide). It is associated with hepatitis B and alcoholic cirrhosis, but can occur without either. It is 10X commoner in men. It presents as pain or a painless swelling. Without treatment the median survival is only 6 months, although 10% will survive 3 years.

Surgical resection offers a chance of cure for localized disease, but recurrence is common. After surgery for small tumours 60% will survive 5 years. The results of liver transplantation are very poor, with a high operative mortality and a high recurrence rate.

Recurrent disease, or inoperable disease, can cause ascites or IVC thrombosis. Hypercalcaemia can occur. Metastases occur to lung and bone.

Chemotherapy produces tumour regression on CT scan in about 20% and can prolong life from a median of 6 months to 2 years. Radiotherapy has no place. Other palliative methods that have been used include transcatheter arterial liver embolization and percutaneous injection of alcohol.

Advanced hepatoma causes liver pain, which responds well to morphine but sometimes requires a coeliac plexus block (*see Nerve blocks*).

Rare complications of hepatoma include: hypercalcaemia, polycythaemia, carcinoid syndrome (wheezing, flushing), ectopic ACTH and hypogylcaemia.

HICCUP

Hiccups are caused by diaphragmatic spasms. The main causes are gastric distension, liver enlargement, malignant mediastinal nodes (causing phrenic nerve irritation) and uraemia. Rarely it can be centrally caused by a brain tumour. Phrenic nerve block is not usually helpful because intercostal spasms continue.

Treatment options are:

- Pharyngeal stimulation (gargling etc.)
- High-dose metoclopramide, 20-30mg QID
- Chlorpromazine 25mg I.V. if severe
- Radiotherapy to mediastinal nodes
- Baclofen 10–20 mg TID
- Anticonvulsant (phenytoin, valproate, carbamazepine)

Reference:
Howard RS. Persistent Hiccups. Br. Med. J. 1992; 305: 1237–8

HOARSENESS

Hoarseness of the voice is usually due to a recurrent laryngeal nerve palsy, due to compression of the nerve by mediastinal nodes or a hilar tumour.

Recurrent laryngeal nerve palsy usually starts suddenly and is painless. The patient can be reassured that the voice will not disappear altogether. It can be treated with a teflon injection if the patient is reasonably well.

Teflon injection is performed by an ENT surgeon. The teflon is injected lateral to the paralysed cord, pushing it medially so that it opposes again with the cord that is still functioning. This can restore the voice to normal.

Laryngeal thrush is a rarer cause, usually associated with inhaled steroids. It can be difficult to eradicate, requiring prolonged systemic anti-fungal therapy (*see Thrush*).

HORMONE THERAPY

Hormone therapy is used to treat recurrent disease in hormone-sensitive tumours: i.e. breast and prostate. It is also occasionally tried for cancer of the kidney and endometrium. Hormone therapy is not curative but can produce excellent palliation of symptoms in some patients. 10% of patients get longterm survival, with no progression of the disease for some years. Cancer cells eventually become independent of the effects of hormone manipulation.

Breast Cancer responds to hormone manipulation in 45% of patients. No clear guidelines exist for the optimum use of hormones in breast cancer. Treatment options include:

- Oophorectomy (pre-menopausal)
- Tamoxifen
- Aminoglutethamide
- Progestagens (medroxyprogesterone or megestrol)
- GnRH analogues

Many patients who respond to tamoxifen will have a second response to aminoglutethamide or medroxyprogesterone.

A response means regression of lesions or the disease becoming static. A response takes 4-8 weeks to occur. A response is more likely in patients over 60 or if there has been a long disease-free interval before recurrence occured. Survival is prolonged if there is a response, to a median of 3 years. The hormone preparation is changed if the disease progresses or if side-effects occur. A response is most easily assessed if there are skin nodules. Bone and lung metastases respond better than brain or liver metastases. As well as improving survival, a response will also reduce symptoms such as local infiltration, enlarged nodes, bone pain, ascites, pleural effusions or hypercalcaemia.

Tamoxifen (Nolvadex) is an oestrogen antagonist and is first-line treatment (cheap, effective). 30-60% respond. The dose is 40mg daily. It has an equivalent effect to oophorectomy. Side-effects include amenorrhoea (in pre-menopausal women), vaginal bleeding, nausea and fluid retention (rarely). A "flare" reaction (bone pain, hypercalcaemia) can occur and is a sign of a response occuring. Patients who initially respond to tamoxifen should receive second-line hormone treatment when the disease starts to progress again.

Aminoglutethimide (Orimeten), in a dose of 250mg daily, increasing to QID is second-line treatment to tamoxifen. It effectively causes a "medical adrenalectomy" and inhibits adrenal oestrogen secretion. Therefore replacement steroids are needed (hydrocortisone 20mg BD). Side-effects include rash and fever (often around day 10) for a few days, and this is self-limiting so the drug should not be stopped. 10% experience nausea and dizziness.

Progestagens are second or third line therapy after tamoxifen. Megestrol acetate (Megace) 160mg daily (single tablet available) or medroxyprogesterone acetate (MPA) (Farlutal, Provera), 200-500mg BD are both used. They have an anti-androgen action and reduce FSH levels. Start with a high dose, e.g. MPA 500mg BD and reduce if side-effects occur. It may improve appetite. Side-effects include fluid retention, flushing, sweats, tremor when the dose should be reduced.

Prostatic cancer responds to hormone manipulation in 80% of cases. Huggins demonstrated a response to oestrogens in 1941. The modern aim is to suppress plasma androgen levels to those found in castrated men, with the fewest possible side-effects. Plasma testosterone levels fall to a tenth of normal with:

- Castration
- GnRH analogues
- Cyproterone 100mg TID
- Oestrogens 1-3mg daily

All these tend to cause impotence and hot flushes. Oestrogens should be avoided because of their cardiovascular side-effects.

GnRH analogues are as effective as orchidecomy and include goserelin (Zoladex) and leuprorelin (Prostap SR), both given by monthly injection.

Flutamide (Drogenil) 250mg TID, blocks adrenal androgen synthesis. It is given for 3 days before starting GnRH analogues, to prevent a flare reaction. The flare is due to initial release of LH before block of the LH receptors occurs. Total suppression of testosterone requires both GnRH analogues and flutamide. Response to hormone therapy can be monitored by Prostate Specific Antigen (PSA). Levels are elevated in cancer to 20–150 microgram\L. Suppression below 10 mcg\L indicates a good response to hormones.

Reference:
Wood BC. Hormone treatments in the common "hormone dependent" carcinomas. Palliative Medicine 1993; 7: 257–272

HOSPICE CARE

A hospice provides multidisciplinary team care that aims to meet the complex and changing needs of a patient and family facing mortal illness. It offers:

- Symptom control
- Rehabilitation
- Respite admissions
- Terminal Care
- Outpatient support
- Family Counselling
- Day care
- Bereavement follow-up

A hospice team usually consists of nurses, doctors, therapists (physiotherapy, OT), social worker, chaplain and volunteers and sometimes a psychologist or counsellor and various complementary therapists.

The need for multi-disciplinary team care is emphasised by looking at patient's concerns. An Australian study of 259 inpatients with cancer (MacAdam, 1987) asked the question "What are your main concerns at present?". The answers were as follows:

CONCERN	HOW OFTEN MENTIONED
Regaining health	45 %
Religion\Philosophy of life	22 %
Concern for spouse	19 %
Concern for children	12 %
Confidence in doctors	7.7 %
Pain relief	5.4 %
Anxiety about treatment	5.4 %
Loss of independence	4.6 %
To get home again	4.2 %
To help others	3.9 %
Effects of treatment	3.0 %
Thoughts of dying	2.3 %
To die peacefully	1.9 %

Hospice nursing should be based on a patient advocacy model, where the nurse's role is to act as the patient's agent and to protect the patient's autonomy, thus restoring control to the patient. The medical model of the nurse being responsible for carrying out the doctor's instructions is not appropriate.

A sense of security is often the key element provided by a hospice team. Once symptoms are controlled and practical needs are met a patient can be released to address some of the other elements of their distress. For some the inner turmoil is so great that they fear they are going mad, and the fear of madness is often greater than the fear of death. A hospice team is able to hold these situations and allow a patient and family the space to adjust to what is happening to them, confident that the team will be able to confidently handle whatever reactions occur.

Comfort care in a hospice setting includes an awareness of the benefits of the following:

- Syringing ear wax
- New optical prescriptions
- Dental care
- Re-lining loose dentures
- Chiropody
- Hairdressing\Manicure

Hospice day care is very supportive for some patients at a certain stage of their illness, especially if they want to remain as independent as possible, but need some help, such as having a weekly bath. Day care is also a good way of supporting carers or introducing a patient who lives alone to a hospice team, before the time they may need terminal care. Many day units also provide opportunities for patients to be creative, or join in with group activities and to remain as active as possible. Patients in this situation also derive a lot of support from each other. To quote Vicky Clement-Jones, who was a doctor and cancer patient (and founder of BACUP), "...we shared our experiences....I realized that other patients could give me something unique which I could not obtain from my doctors or nurses, however caring".

References:
Stedeford A. Hospice – a safe place to suffer? Palliative Medicine 1987; 1. 73-74.
MacAdam DB, Smith M. An initial assessment of suffering in terminal illness. Palliative Medicine 1987; 1: 37-47.
Webber J, Accountability, advocacy and the nurse. Palliative Medicine 1987; 1: 53-56.

HYPERCALCAEMIA

Hypercalcaemia is defined as a serum calcium above 2.6 mmol\l. Hypercalcaemia causes unpleasant symptoms. Above 4.0mmol\l it will cause death in a few days if untreated.

The corrected calcium level allows for hypoproteinaemia: add 0.02mmol\l to the serum calcium level for every 1g\l of albumin below 40.

The prevalence of hypercalcaemia is about 10% of cancer patients. It can occur at any stage in the disease and most episodes are mild and self-limiting. In a survey of patients with breast cancer who had calcium levels measured every 6 weeks, 43% developed mild hypercalcaemia at some time. In a prospective hospice survey of cancer patients who had calcium measured on admission, only 17 out of 200 (8.5%) were found to have corrected calcium levels above 2.7mmol\l, only 6 had levels above 3.0mmol\l, and only 2 had levels above 4.0mmol\l. (Lancet 2 March 1985, page 512).

Malignant causes of hypercalcaemia are most commonly cancers of the bronchus (squamous) and breast, and haematological malignancies (especially myeloma, but also lymphoma and leukaemia).

Cancers of the bronchus and breast account for 50% of cases of hypercalcaemia. Myeloma is a rarer disease but 30% develop hypercalcaemia. Squamous cancers of the head and neck and oesophagus and genito-urinary cancers (renal, cervix, uterus, ovary) can all cause hypercalcaemia.

Hypercalcaemia is very rare with adenocarcinomas of the stomach, colon and prostate (even with extensive bone metastases) and does not occur in adenocarcinoma or small cell cancer of the lung.

Non-malignant causes of hypercalcaemia are occasionally relevant. It can occur after tamoxifen is started as part of a flare reaction (*see Hormones*) and in vitamin D intoxication. If hypercalcaemia occurs in a patient with a history of cancer and if there is no other evidence of recurrent disease, it is important to exclude primary hyperparathyroidism (which is curable by excising benign parathyroid adenomas), by measuring Parathormone levels, which are high and diagnostic, being low in malignant hypercalcaemia.

Symptoms of hypercalcaemia include loss of energy, muscle weakness, drowsiness, nausea, vomiting, constipation, polyuria, polydipsia, confusion and coma. In advanced cancer hypercalcaemia is often mild and asymptomatic, and symptoms usually only develop with levels above 3.0 mmol\l. Hypercalcaemia should be particularly susupected if there is:

- Drowsiness
- Nausea and vomiting
- Thirst

In the hospice survey of hypercalcaemia mentioned above, there were fewer symptoms than expected. 9 out of the 17 cases (53%) had moderate or severe drowsiness, but only 3 had severe nausea and vomiting, and only 2 had thirst, the 2 with calcium levels above 4.0mmol\l.

The mechanism of hypercalcaemia is due to the secretion of a tumour peptide called parathormone releasing protein (PTHrH). This causes both increased calcium release from bone (osteoclastic activity) and decreased excretion of calcium in urine. Bone metastases (even extensive bone metastases) alone are not enough to cause hypercalcaemia if renal excretion is normal. Elevated PTHrH levels have been identified in a variety of human tumours including lung, breast, kidney and skin. PTHrH is immunologically distinct from normal PTH, which is never elevated in malignancy.

Prognosis tends to be poor with hypercalcaemia of malignancy (80% survive less than one year). However, some cancer patients, especially with breast cancer, can have a self-limiting episode of hypercalcaemia early in the course of their disease, which may go undetected or which after treatment does not recur.

Treatment is only necessary if there are symptoms, and lowering calcium levels may not be indicated if the patient is close to death. Treatment involves both rehydration and lowering of calcium levels, and the biphosphonates are now the mainstay of treatment.

- Fluids
- IV pamidronate
- Oral clodronate
- Calcitonin
- Steroids
- Hormone therapy

Oral fluids are often sufficient to control mild hypercalcaemia with calcium levels around 2.6-3.0 mmol\l. Encourage oral fluids and monitor calcium levels.

IV fluids may be needed for calcium levels above 3.0 mmol\l, if the patient is dehydrated. High volumes of fluid are not necessary and risk causing fluid overload. Give 2-3 litres of Normal saline over 24 hours, then 2 litres a day until rehydrated. Potassium supplements are usually needed. Calcium levels will only fall 0.1-0.4 mmol\l as a result of IV fluids, and pamidronate will usually be needed as well.

Pamidronate (Aredia) is the treatment of choice for severe hypercalcaemia. It is a biphosphonate and a potent osteoclast inhibitor. It has the advantage that a single infusion every 3 weeks can normalize calcium levels and is therefore preferred to etidronate. Studies show it is effective in 70-90% for an average of 20-30 days. The initial dose is 30mg, added to 500ml of Normal saline and given over 4 hours. Each additional 15mg require at least 125ml of saline over 2 hours, up to a maximum of 90mg for a single treatment. The calcium levels starts to fall after 48 hours and gradually fall for the next 6 days. Depending on the calcium levels, subsequent doses may need to be higher, (maximum 90mg per treatment). It should be withheld if serum creatine is above 250 micromol\l until the patient has been rehydrated for 24-48 hours, as there have been reports of renal impairment caused by biphosphonates. 25% of patients develop a transient pyrexia for 24 hours after infusion. Monitor calcium levels weekly.

Clodronate (Loron) is an oral biphosphonate that is reported to be effective in delaying the recurrence of hypercalcaemia. The dose is 400mg 6 hourly, increasing to 800mg 6 hourly if necessary. It is used to maintain normal calcium levels after severe or recurrent hypercalcaemia. It is very poorly absorbed and if taken with food or milky drinks none at all is absorbed. It can cause nausea. It is expensive.

Calcitonin has the advantage that it lowers calcium levels quickly (by acting on both bone and kidney) but it only causes a modest fall in calcium levels, and the effect only lasts 2-3 days. It is best given with steroids, which enhance the effect. Give Salcatonin (Calsynar) SC 200 units 8 hourly (6 hourly if severe), with oral dexamethasone 8mg per day. It tends to cause nausea, vomiting and sometimes facial flushing. It is expensive.

Steroids have a reputation for lowering calcium levels, probably dating back to an enthusiastic report in 1965 by Mannheimer. However later studies have all shown that steroids are almost always ineffective in solid tumours. Steroids <u>will</u> lower calcium levels in myeloma and lymphomas (and possibly some types of breast and renal cancer, where the mechanism of hypercalcaemia is probably different to other solid tumours). Even when efffective, steroids take several days to be effective and their effect is usually only partial.

Hormone therapy can prevent the recurrence of hypercalcaemia in hormone-sensitive breast cancer.

Other treatments are rarely needed. Low dietary calcium is unnecessary because calcium absorbtion is already low in cancer patients. Oral phosphate (phosphate-Sandoz) 500mg TID will reduce calcium levels, and was the only orally effective treatment prior to the arrival of clodronate, but it can cause severe diarrhoea. IV phosphate will reduce severe hypercalcaemia within 24 hours, but has been associated with sudden deaths and is rarely used. IV Plicamycin (mithramycin) is less used now as the effect only lasts about a week and side-effects are more common than with pamidronate. Other treatments that have been used include gallium nitrate, trisodium edetate, octreotide and peritoneal dialysis.

Further reading:
Heath DA. Review article: Hypercalcaemia in malignancy. Palliative Medicine. 1989; 3: 1-11.

INSOMNIA

Insomnia means poor quality sleep. It can cause great distress to the patient, worsens most symptoms and can exhaust carers so that they can no longer cope. A good night's sleep brings a great deal of comfort.

The cause of insomnia may be reversible. Anxiety and depression both seem worse at night. There may be a physical cause such as:

- Pain
- Stiffness
- Cramps
- Sweating
- Incontinence

Drug treatment of insomnia may require temazepam, chlorpromazine or amitriptyline.

Temazepam, 10-60mg, is suitable for most patients, provided the correct dose is used. Some patients sleep poorly even on 60mg, and require nitrazepam instead, others are over-sedated even on 10mg temazepam, when chlormethiazole (Heminevrin) or zopiclone should be used instead, especially in the confused and elderly. Diazepam is only used if a long-acting anxiolytic effect is required. Tolerance develops to all the benzodiazepines within 2-3 weeks, if given every night.

Zopiclone (Zimovane) is a cyclopyrrolone which is said to cause less dependence and less morning hangover of drowsiness. 7.5mg is the usual dose. Half-lives of the commonly used hypnotics are given in the table.

Chlorpromazine, 25-50mg is useful if anxiety is causing insomnia, and potentiates other hynotics. if evening anxiety occurs, doses of chlorpromazine can be given at 6pm and bed time, together with temazepam.

Amitriptyline, 25-150mg, is useful if a sedative anti-depressant is required, and will also potentiate temazepam.

HALF-LIVES OF HYPNOTICS	
HYPNOTIC DRUG	HALF-LIFE (hours)
Long-acting hypnotics	
Flurazepam (Dalmane)	47-95
Diazepam	21-46
Nitrazepam (Mogadon)	18-36
Flunitrazepam (Rohypnol)	22
Short-acting hypnotics	
Zopiclone(Zimovane)	4-7
Temazepam	5-11
Lormetazepam	10
Chloral hydrate (Welldorm)	7-10
Chlormethiazole(Heminevrin)	4-5

Intractable insomnia is very distressing. If the patient is not sleeping with the above medication a useful treatment is an I.M. injection of the combination of drugs below, which usually ensures good quality sleep for at least 4 hours and can be repeated if necessary.

- Diamorphine 2.5-5mg (if the patient is already on morphine, the dose may need to be higher)
- Chlorpromazine 50mg
- Hyoscine 0.4mg

INTERVENTIONAL RADIOLOGY

Interventional radiology includes the following techniques:

- Hepatic artery embolization
- Renal artery embolization
- Internal iliac artery embolization
- Biliary drainage (external or internal)
- Percutaneous nephrostomy
- IVC filter
- SVC stents

Hepatic artery embolization is occasionally used for liver pain or to reduce the hormone production from carcinoid metastases (flushing, wheezing) or insulin-secreting metastases (hypoglycaemia). A catheter is inserted into the hepatic artery, via the aorta and coeliac artery. The circulation is then blocked, one method being to inject gelatin sponge, which blocks the smaller peripheral arteries and then to insert a metal coil, which blocks the main artery. The procedure is only performed if the portal venous flow is intact, so that total liver necrosis does not occur, and if the arterial supply is distorted or abberant it is not always possible. It is followed by tissue necrosis, with severe pain and fever for 2-5 days, (post-embolization syndrome) which requires high dose morphine. The technique demands radiological skill in arterial catheterization, which may atrophy with the advent of magnetic resonance angiography.

Renal artery embolization can control bleeding or pain from inoperable renal tumours. The tumour can re-vascularize over a period of months and the procedure can then be repeated.

Internal iliac artery embolization can be used to control bleeding from pelvic tumours. There is a small risk of bladder necrosis.

Biliary drainage is usually performed now by the insertion of a stent by an endoscopist. Self-expanding metal stents are available. When stent insertion is not possible and the patient is troubled with severe itching, bile can be drained by inserting a catheter externally, via the percutanous transhepatic route. The catheter may pass through the obstruction, so that some bile drains internally into the duodenum, or the bile may all pass externally, where it is collected into a stoma bag (and tends to leak and make a mess – which can be reduced by putting absorbtion flakes into the bag, which draws the bile down into the bag to form a gel with the flakes). The main problem is cholangitis, and antibiotics should be started promptly if fever develops.

Percutaneous nephrostomy is a simple technique to perform if there is obstructive uropathy causing renal failure or pain. The dilated renal pelvis lies close to the surface, and a catheter is easily inserted, avoiding renal arteries. It is connected to a urine bag which can be worn on the leg. It can be changed to a permanent surgical nephrostomy at a later date, if necessary.

IVC filters can be inserted in a patient with recurrent pulmonary emboli. It is a relatively simple procedure and should be considered if anti-coagulation is proving ineffective or is contra-indicated.

SVC stents may become available to treat some cases of SVC compression (*see SVCO*).

INTESTINAL OBSTRUCTION

Intestinal obstruction typically causes abdominal distension, colic, vomiting and absolute constipation (no motions or wind). Malignant intestinal obstruction occurs in 3% of hospice patients. It can differ from the classic picture in several ways. There may be little abdominal distension, if widespread tumour infiltration has occured. It may be episodic and may occur for a few days and then settle down, and diarrhoea may occur as well as constipation, because it is due to a dysfunction of the bowel, rather than a straightforward mechanical obstruction.

Causes of malignant intestinal obstruction are most commonly cancers of the ovary (25%) and colo-rectum (10%) but occasionally other tumours (including uterus, prostate, bladder, stomach and lymphoma).

Diagnosis can be confirmed by a plain abdominal X-ray (supine and erect) which may show dilated loops of bowel or fluid levels in the bowel (on the erect film). However, if the bowel is full of fluid it will not show on X-ray, but will show on real-time ultrasound scan.

Management options for intestinal obstruction include:

- Surgery
- NG suction\IV fluids
- Symptom control by subcutaneous drugs

Surgery must be considered for any cancer patient developing intestinal obstruction for the first time. 10% will have a benign cause, 10% will have another primary, and many will be amenable to palliative surgery to relieve the obstruction. However, if obstruction recurs, medical management is usually a better option than further surgery, which is only considered if there is good evidence of a single block in a relatively fit patient.

Nasogastric suction and IV fluids is standard pre-operative management, but it is not appropriate for prolonged inoperable obstruction.

Nasogastric suction is only indicated in advanced cancer for the severe, distressing vomiting of high obstruction. This pattern of vomiting can settle with high dose steroids (dexamenthasone 8mg) in about 50% of cases and the tube can then be removed.

IV fluids are only indicated if the patient is complaining of thirst, which is unusual.

A subcutaneous infusion of drugs can control symptoms. A common combination of drugs, mixed together in the syringe driver and infused over 24 hours is:

- Diamorphine (50% of 24 hour oral morphine)
- Buscopan 60mg (for colic)
- Cyclizine 150mg (for nausea)

See also Subcutaneous Infusions.

High dose steroids (dexamethasone 8mg per 24 hours) may increase the chance of the obstruction resolving. In a small double-blind cross-over trial of 21 patients, dexamethasone seemed to increase the chance of the obstruction resolving:

	OBSTRUCTION RESOLVED	
	YES	NO
Dexamethasone	9	4
Placebo	4	4

The aim of treatment is to control symptoms and to allow eating and drinking. Patients with obstruction can drink fluids and keep themselves well hydrated for weeks using this regime. An oral bowel softener (but not a stimulant laxative) should be given daily. Intravenous fluids are only needed if the patient is thirsty (which is unusual).

Vomiting is the most difficult symptom to control, and about a third of these patients will continue to vomit. This is usually well tolerated if the nausea is abolished and the aim of the treatment is explained.

Octreotide (Sandostatin) has a place in the control of intractable obstructive vomiting. In a study of 14 patients with malignant bowel obstruction, an SC infusion of octreotide, 300–600 micrograms per 24 hours, controlled vomiting in 12 patients (Mercadante *et al*, 1993). Octreotide inhibits hormone release and reduces both gastro-intestinal motility and secretions. In one case study, a patient with a nasogastric tube had greatly reduced aspirates, from 1-2 litres to 300ml per day. (Reference: Khoo D *et al*, Lancet 8 February 1992, p 375-6.)

Post-mortem examination of 18 hospice patients with malignant intestinal obstruction (8 ovary, 7 large bowel) showed most had extrinsic compression at multiple levels from adhesions and masses, although 4 had a single site of obstruction. The bowel was often seeded with tumour deposits and long segments of gut were stiff and congested (possibly explaining the episodes of diarrhoea that can occur). Only 1 patient had peritonitis. The median survival was suprisingly long, at 3.7 months (Baines *et al*, 1985).

Reference:
Baines M, Oliver DJ, Carter RL, Medical management of intestinal obstruction in patients with advanced malignant disease – a clinical and pathological study, Lancet 2 November 1985 p 990-993.
Mercadante S. *et al*. Octreotide in relieving gastro-intestinal symptoms due to bowel obstruction. Palliative Medicine 1993; 7: 295–299

ITCH

Itch (pruritus) is a form of pain. There is no generally effective anti-pruritic. Itching is usually due to jaundice or is a secondary to the malignancy. Rarer causes are <u>allergies</u> (especially to new soaps or perfumes) and <u>scabies</u> (AIDS patients can have dramatic infestations with scabies before itching occurs).

General advice is to avoid overheating which increases itch. Avoid hot baths and wear cotton cloths. The <u>first step</u> in treatment is to get the patient sleeping well, either with temazepam 10-60mg, or sedative anti-histamines, or both.

Drug reactions usually cause a generalized rash as well as itching, but <u>chlorpromazine</u> can cause cholestasis, with itching, and jaundice may not be clinically obvious.

Jaundice causes itch because bile acids are absorbed into the circulation and skin. Jaundice may cause severe itching that merits biliary drainage (*see Jaundice*).

Antihistamines. <u>Terfenadine</u> (Triludan) 60mg BD, or the forte tablet (120mg) daily, or suspension (30mg\5ml) is one of the newer non-sedative antihistamines. It can help in all types of itching, including jaundice. It has been associated with arrythmias in high dosage, and should not be given with erythromcyin or ketoconazole, which inhibit its metabolism.

<u>Other non-sedative anti-histamines</u> include astemizole (Hismanal), cetirizine (Zirtek) and loratadine (Clarityn). Sometimes a sedative anti-histamine is

more helpful, such as chlorpheniramine (Piriton) 4mg 4 hourly, or 12mg at night. Other sedating anti-histamines include cyproheptadine (Periactin), promethazine (Phenergan), trimeprazine (Vallergan), azatadine (Optimine) and brompheniramine (Dimotane).

Creams that can reduce itching include:

- Calamine
- Crotamiton
- Oilatum
- Topical steroids

Calamine lotion is soothing, cooling the skin by evaporation, and leaving a fine coating of powder.

Crotamiton (Eurax), cream or lotion, is effective for some patients. Avoid the eyes.

Oilatum emollient bath additive, 5-15ml per bath (cool), is a useful hydrating agent for the dry skin; soak for 10-20 minutes.

Topical steroids are helpful if scratching has caused secondary inflammation.

Plasma exchange has been used as a last resort to relieve severe itching in some situations, including lymphoma.

JAUNDICE

Jaundice means yellow staining of the skin and eyes due to obstruction to the flow of bile. Bile fails to reach the bowel (so motions are pale) and is forced into the circulation (dark urine).

In cancer patients the cause of jaundice is usually malignant obstruction to the common bile duct by a primary tumour (pancreas, bile duct) or enlarged nodes at the porta hepatis. Jaundice is very rarely due to liver metastases alone. Jaundice itself does not shorten the prognosis, and some patients live some months.

The main symptom of jaundice is itch, which is an indication for treatment. Itch from jaundice may be severe in one patient, and none occur at all in another. Sometimes it is not possible to abolish itching, when it may be helpful for the patient to know that for unknown reasons the itching can settle or disappear after a time (usually weeks) even though the jaundice persists. Itch is a form of pain and biliary drainage should always be considered. Itch in jaundice may not respond to specific measures and may be helped by antihistamines and creams (*see Itch*).

Medical treatments for itching due to jaundice include:

- Exchange resin
- Steroids (to relieve biliary pressure)
- Stanozolol 5-10mg daily

Exchange resins can reduce itching if there is partial blockage to bile drainage, by binding to bile acids in the gut and preventing their reabsorbtion into the circulation. They are not effective if there is total obstruction. They include cholestyramine (Questran) and colestipol (Colestid), which is more palatable. Colestipol 5-10g BD is taken with water (sachet of yellow granules). It can cause nausea and flatulence. It should be taken 1 hour before other medication, to reduce possible interference with drug absorbtion.

High dose steroids may reduce pressure on the bile duct by reducing peri-tumour oedema.

Stanozolol (Stromba) 5-10mg daily can sometimes reduce itching in obstructive jaundice. It is an anabolic steroid and the mechanism of action in itching is unknown. Paradoxically it has the rare side-effect of causing cholestatic jaundice.

Biliary obstruction can be confirmed by ultrasound scan, which shows dilated ducts. Absence of dilated ducts means the obstruction is occuring in the liver, possibly due to a drug reaction (most commonly chlorpromazine). Methods of biliary drainage include:

- Surgical drainage of bile (cholecystojejunostomy)
- Biliary stent
- External bile drainage

Cholecystjcjunostomy is performed whenever possible if cancer of the head of pancreas is found at laparotomy. Stents are inserted into the bile duct via the duodenum and ampulla of Vater by endoscopy, when low obstructions can often be overcome by internal stenting. Stenting may not be possible with high obstructions when external drainage can be considered. A percutaneous transhepatic catheter can be passed by a radiologist, but this leaves the patient with a tube draining bile externally, which brings its own problems of skin soreness and leaking onto clothing (*see Interventional Radiology*).

Radiotherapy may be helpful if there are enlarged nodes (seen on CT scan) compressing the bile duct.

LASERS

A laser is a sophisticated light source. Einstein first proposed the concept of stimulated light emission in 1917. LASER stands for Light Amplification by

Stimulated Emission of Radiation. It was invented in 1960 and the carbon dioxide laser was first used medically in 1967. There are 3 main types in medical use:

- CO_2 laser – cervix
- Argon laser – skin, eye
- Nd YAG laser – tumour palliation

The Nd YAG laser (ND YAG means neodymium yttrium-aluminium-garnet) was first used medically in 1977 to treat bleeding lesions in the upper GI tract. In 1982 it was used to palliate dysphagia due to oesophageal cancers. It is a more powerful laser, and yet the beam of light is still narrow enough to be transmitted by 0.5mm fibres, and so it can be used via a firbeoptic endoscope. Tumours can be vapourized and coagulated and haemorrhage from vessels up to 1mm diameter can be controlled.

Relief of symptoms can be immediate, with no side-effects, but may involve repeated endoscopy. Laser treatment can:

- Re-canalize tumours
- Debulk tumours
- Control haemorrhage

It can control symptoms such as dysphagia, dyspnoea due to an obstructing bronchial tumour, haemoptysis, rectal bleeding or obstruction. It can be especially useful for the urgent treatment of tracheal tumours causing stridor.

Interstitial laser hyperthermia can be used to cause tumour necrosis for tumours in organs that are difficult to resect, such as liver and pancreas. It is delivered at low power (1-2 Watts rather that 60-80 Watts) via needles inserted directly into the tumour. Precise areas of necrosis up to 5cm diameter can be produced which heal safely. Treatment of hollow organs, such as colon or bladder risks later perforation.

Photodynamic therapy can cause tumour necrosis. It involves the laser activation of a photo-sensitizer that is retained by cancer cells. A photo-sensitizer (photofrin) is given which is concentrated by tumour cells, and 2 days later is activated by laser light, which releases oxygen and destroys tumour cells. Light can only penetrate 10mm into living tissues, limiting the technique. It may have a useful place in palliation, by reducing tumour bulk, and may come to have a place in the primary treatment of small tumours of the bronchus, bladder and GI tract and head and neck. It can be used externally or interstitially or for any lesions accessible to light via endoscope, laparoscope or percutaneous (ultrasound-guided) route or for retrobulbar tumours.

Further Reading:
The British Journal of Hospital Medicine vol 40, Sept 1988 has a series of articles on the medical uses of lasers.
Hetzel MR. Laser palliation of tracheobronchial tumours: a review. Palliative Medicine 1988; 2: 134-8.

LAXATIVES

Laxatives are drugs that ease defaecation. The commonly used laxatives in the hospice setting are:

- Lactulose
- Senna
- Co-danthramer
- Co-danthrusate
- Bisacodyl

Lactulose with senna is more effective than normal strength co-danthramer. A randomized cross-over study of 58 hospice patients showed that mean stool frequency with lactulose and senna (4.2 motions per week) was significantly higher than with co-danthramer (mean 2.5 per week). Doses were titrated to individual response. The need for rectal measures was also higher with co-danthramer (37% of patients – the hospice average) than with lactulose and senna (18%). The dose of laxative needs to be titrated in ALL patients on opoids. There is statistically no significant difference in laxative doses needed by patients on high or low dose morphine (Sykes 1991).

The pharmacology of laxatives is complex and remains poorly understood. They can be classified into softeners, stimulants and bulking agents. Softeners include unabsorbed sugars (lactulose), unabsorbed salts (magnesium sulphate), surface-wetting agents (docustate) and lubricants (liquid paraffin). Stimulants include polyphenolics (bisacodyl, sodium picosulphate) and anthraquinones (Senna, danthron). Bulking agents include ispaghula (fybogel, isogel, regulan) and sterculia (normocol).

Clinically useful laxatives are listed in the table. Most patients require a combination of a softener and a stimulant laxative.

Lactulose (Duphalac) syrup is a non-absorbed sugar, galactose-fructose (safe for diabetics). It causes water to be retained in the bowel. 30ml increases stool volume by 500ml, which stimulates peristalsis. 20-40ml are needed BD, with a stimulant laxative for most patients on opioids. It takes 2-3 days to take effect. Tolerance may develop, so higher doses are needed after a time. 20% complain of wind and distension (gut bacteria metabolize the sugars) and some find it too sweet.

Liquid paraffin is a lubricant and softener, and is useful for patients who dislike lactulose. It is best given as liquid paraffin and magnesium hydroxide mixture (Milpar) 5-20ml BD. Too much can cause a leak of liquid paraffin from the anus.

Docusate sodium (Dioctyl), tablets or syrup, 100-500mg daily is a mild softening agent, allowing water to penetrate the stool, and also slightly increases gut secretions. It is not effective alone for most patients on opioids.

TABLE OF USEFUL LAXATIVES

Softeners:

- Lactulose (Duphalac)
- Docusate (Dioctyl) tablets or syrup
- Liquid paraffin and magnesium hydroxide (Milpar)

Stimulants:

- Senna tablets or syrup
- Bisacodyl (Dulcolax) tablets
- Picosulphate (Picolax) sachet
- Magnesium sulphate

Bulking agents:

- Fybogel (ispaghula) sachets
- Normacol (sterculia) teaspoons

Combined stimulant plus softener

- Co-danthramer (Codalax) suspension
- Co-danthrusate (Normax) capsules

CONTENT OF COMBINED LAXATIVES

	Danthron	Poloxamer	Docusate
Co-danthramer (5ml) (Codalax suspen.)	25mg	200mg	-
Co-danthramer forte (5ml) (Codalax forte)	75mg	1000mg	–
Co-danthrusate (Normax capsule)	50mg	–	60mg

N.B. Danthron (in co-danthramer and co-danthrusate) stains urine red.

Stimulant laxatives are effective within 6-12 hours. They are contact agents and act directly on the bowel wall to increase peristalsis. (In experiments, local anaesthetic applied to the bowel abolishes their effect). Abdominal cramps can occur. They include:

- Co-danthramer (or forte) 5-25ml BD
- Co-danthrusate capsules 1-6 BD
- Senna tablets, 1-4, B.D.
- Bisacodyl (Dulcolax) 5-10mg, B.D.

- Picosulphate (Picolax sachet, 1 in the morning)
- Magnesium sulphate

Bulking agents alone are not effective in preventing constipation in patients on opioids. They produce a soft formed stool and are useful in anal fissures, colostomy management, and to control the discharge in rectal cancers. The effect can take several days to develop. They should be taken with plenty of water and avoided if there is any risk of obstruction.

- Bran (not usually tolerated)
- Fybogel 1-2 sachets a day
- Normacol 1-2 5ml teaspoons a day

Magnesium sulphate is an unabsorbed salt, a saline flusher, retaining water in the bowel, and also stimulates peristalsis. It is effective in 3-6 hours, usually causing diarrhoea. It useful for constipation that is resistant to other laxatives. Magnesium sulphate mixture BP, 10-20ml, is taken in the morning with plenty of water. In patients with renal failure there is a small risk of hypermagnesaemia if used repeatedly, (which can be asymptomatic, but may cause confusion).

Reference:
Sykes NP. A Clinical comparison of laxatives in a hospice. Palliative Medicine 1991; 5: 307-314.

LEUKAEMIAS

Leukaemias cause around 4000 deaths per year in the UK. They are malignancies of white blood cells that infiltrate the bone marrow causing anaemia, thrombocyopenia (bleeding) and agranulocytosis (infections). They also involves lymph tissue (enlarged nodes, hepatosplenomegaly) and other tissues (CNS, bone, skin). Diagnosis is based on finding lymphoblasts in the marrow. Chronic leukaemias occur in the elderly, acute leukaemias at any age. 50% of children and 25% of young adults can be cured.

Chronic lymphatic leukaemia typically causes anaemia, enlarged nodes and repeated chest infections. It is treated with chlorambucil and radiotherapy to enlarged nodes. 50% survive 5 years. Symptomless patients may survive 5-20 years after diagnosis.

Chronic myeloid leukaemia typically causes anaemia and massive enlargement of the liver and spleen. It is treated with Busulphan and 50% survive 3 years. Finally it transforms into an acute leukaemia (blast crisis) which is more aggressive, and even intense chemotherapy can rarely extend life beyond about a year.

Acute myeloid leukaemia is much less responsive to treatment. 80% get a remission with chemotherapy, but cure is rare. Blood transfusion can help even if chemotherapy is inappropriate.

Acute lymphatic leukaemia is the commonest form in chilhood with good cure rates with chemotherapy and cranial irradiation. If relapse occurs intensive treatment with bone marrow transplant is needed to produce a cure.

The terminal phase in leukaemia is often short and painfree, although bone pains and painful splenic infarcts can occur. Platelet transfusions may still be considered for distressing bleeding (retinal, nose). Chemotherapy may still be appropriate if CNS disease is causing distressing symptoms.

LUNG CANCER

Lung Cancer causes 40,000 deaths per year, more than any other cancer, and is the commonest cancer in men. It is strongly associated with smoking, but 15% occur in non-smokers (usually adenocarinomas). Presentation may be with cough, haemoptysis, dyspnoea, chest pains or wheeze.

Small-cell lung cancer accounts for 15-20% of lung cancer. It disseminates early and widely (to bone, liver, lymphatics and brain) but responds to chemotherapy, which can prolong survival. When the disease is still localized, chemotherapy can prolong survival to 2 years in 15-20%, and 5 years for 5%. With advanced disease chemotherapy can prolong survival from a median of 2 to 9 months, but most patients have died within 18 months. 30% develop brain metastases even after chemotherapy.

Non-small cell lung cancers (squamous, large cell, adeno) can be resected if peripheral and if there are no metastases. 20% are operable and 20% of these are cured. Radiotherapy probably does not prolong survival. Chemotherapy is disappointing and even toxic combinations produce very small response rates, and it remains restricted to clinical trials. Average survival from diagnosis depends on histology, and is around 18 months for squamous and large cell tumuors, and 36 months for adenocarcinomas.

Local spread of lung cancer causes pleural effusions, hilar node enlargement, pericardial involvement (effusion, arrhythmias) and enlarged mediastinal nodes with compression of the SVC, oesophagus (dysphagia), laryngeal nerve (*see Hoarseness*), sympathetic chain (ptosis) or phrenic nerve (paralysed diaphragm).

Apical lung tumours can cause Pancoast's syndrome, with arm pain due to damage to the brachial plexus (C8, T1 nerve roots) with severe pain in the medial side of the arm, and damage to the sympathetic nerves causes Horner's syndrome with ptosis, a drooping eyelid, a small pupil and absent sweating on the same side of the face. 5% get vertebral spread and cord compression. Radiotherapy can control pain in 80%. Survival after treatment is 9-48 months.

Palliative radiotherapy for lung cancer is useful in 50% to control symptoms by shrinking the tumour or mediastinal nodes (causing dysphagia, SVCO or stridor). Haemoptysis responds in 90% cough, dyspnoea and visceral chest pains respond in around 40%. A typical regime is 20Gy in 5 fractions. 17Gy in 2 fractions has been shown to be as effective, but can cause acute radiation oesophagitis. Bone pain from metastases respond in 80% of cases and in long bones can be treated with a single shot (*see Bone pain*).

Non-metastatic manifestations of lung cancer are mostly rare and include:

- Clubbing
- Arthralgia (wrists and ankles)
- Ectopic ACTH
- Hypercalcaemia (20% of squamous cancers)
- SIADH (20% of small cell cancers)
- Neuropathies\myopathies
- Myasthenia (*see Weakness*)
- Thrombophlebitis
- Endocarditis

Problems in advanced cancer of the lung commonly include:

- Pain
- Dyspnoea
- Cough, haemoptysis
- Dysphagia, stridor, SVCO, hoarseness
- Nodal enlargement or ulceration
- Skin nodules
- Hypercalcaemia
- Brain metastases (40%)

Brain metastases are occasionally worth treating with cranial irradiation, especially in adenocarcinomas, when survival can be prolonged from a median of 1 to 5 months and symptoms improved (*see Brain metastases*).

Reference:
Souhami R, Current issues in cancer, Br Med J 1992; 304: 1298-301.

LYMPHOEDEMA

Lymphoedema means swelling of a limb due to damaged deep lymphatics. It is caused by blockage of the lymphatics may be due to malignant cells, radiation fibrosis, surgery or recurrent infections. It occurs in 38% of women with breast cancer after axillary clearance plus RT.

Treatment of lymphoedema aims to:

- Reduce swelling and discomfort
- Improve limb mobility
- Avoid skin damage or cellulitis

Compression therapy is the mainstay of treatment and is usually undertaken by a physiotherapist or nurse. The principle of treatment is that firm compression of the limb can reduce the swelling over a period of weeks. When deep lymphatics are blocked, circulation through the superficial lymphatics must be stimulated. Bandaging has been shown to increase lymph drainage in healthy volunteers, and circulation is further increased by active contraction of muscles while bandaged. Treatment is monitored by measuring the circumference of the limb at several points every week. It may involve:

- Bandaging
- Compression pump
- Elastic support
- Massage and exercises
- Skin care

Bandaging (see below for details) is time-consuming but effective. Bandages are worn for 24 hours a day for approximately 2 weeks. The bandages are renewed daily. It may need to be repeated after 6-8 weeks. It is used to treat severe or long-standing swelling, and in certain special situations where an elastic support garment would be inadequate:

- Awkward-shaped limb
- Pain
- Recurrent bouts of infection
- Lymph leak

Compression pumps (Jobst, Flotron, Talley, Lymphapress) are useful to speed up the inital process of compression, especially in hardened tissues, but do not achieve a better final result than bandaging. Multichamber sequential pumps (Multicom, Centromed) produce a wave of compression starting distally and are most effective but expensive. The Multipulse PT 202 produced by Talley Medical Equipment is a 10 chamber pump with controls for cycle time (30, 70, 110 seconds), treatment time (30 or 60 minutes or continuous) and pressure (60-130mmHg).

The principles of using the pumps are:

- 3 hours a day for 2 weeks
- Pressure up to 60 mm Hg, normally
- Elastic support as well (to maintain effect)
- Avoid if limb is painful
- Avoid in trunk oedema
- Wait 8 weeks after a DVT

Elastic support sleeve or stocking is essential to maintain the improvement gained, and should be worn all day but can be removed at night. Off-the-shelf garments are used until limb size is static, then made-to-measure garments can be bought. Patients too weak to pull on an elastic sleeve or stocking can use a double layer of shaped tubigrip (straight tubigrip that rolls down has the effect of a garter). Elastic compression sleeves and stockings are made by Duomed and Scholl and can be prescribed on FP10, and are made to measure.

Massage of the trunk can reduce swelling of a limb by stimulating lymph flow in the superficial lymph vessels, which normally depends on body movement. If there is swelling of the axillary fold there is trunk oedema. Massage is the only way to shift lymphoedema that involves the trunk, head and neck or genitalia. Fluid is massaged <u>away</u> from the affected site (starting on the <u>opposite</u> side of the trunk to the affected area) for 15 minutes twice a day. An electric body massager can be helpful.

Exercises, active or passive, will reduce swelling and prevent joint stiffness, and should be done with compression support on the limb. <u>Slings</u> should be avoided and only worn if the arm is paralysed, because immobility increases swelling.

Skin care is essential because with severe swelling there is often reduced sensation in the swollen limb and poor skin condition due to reduced circulation, predisposing to skin ulceration. Routine care involves:

- Regular aqueous cream (skin hydration)
- Avoid hard objects (pressure damage)
- Don't risk cuts or scratches
- Use creams (not razors) to remove hair
- Avoid heat or strong detergents
- Avoid sunburn and hot baths
- Use protective gloves (cooking, washing up)
- Avoid procedures (BP, venepuncture) in that arm
- Antibiotics for cellulitis (teach recognition)

Compliance with compression therapy was surveyed in 33 cancer patients with chronic lymphoedema of the arm, and the high compliance suggests the treatment is effective. 97% continued to use a compression sleeve (80% every day), 75% carried out arm exercises, 45% used trunk massage. Only 12% used a compression pump. 80% had continuing trouble finding clothes to fit the arm. Half had pain or reduced arm function. 73% found attendance at the lymphoedema clinic psychologically supportive (Palliative Medicine 1991; 5: 52-55).

Prophylactic antibiotics may be needed on a longterm basis if there has been recurrent cellulitis. Each episode of cellulitis can cause further damage. The arm may be red and inflamed but the infection can be sub-clinical and present simply as worsening swelling or a feeling of malaise. Prophylactic penicillin V 500mg daily may be sufficient, but if the infection persists Flucloxacillin is needed and if it still persists advice from a microbiologist should be sought.

Diuretics are usually ineffective. Early lymphoedema may respond partially to a combination of high-dose steroids and diuretics, and this is worth trying, but is usually ineffective. If there is soft pitting oedema, it suggests a venous component, and a diuretic is then more likely to have an effect (*see Diuretics*).

The Technique of bandaging: Arms and legs are bandaged in a similar way. Three-layer bandage is applied daily Monday to Friday, left for the week-end and applied for another week. Measurements are taken regularly, and if the limb stops reducing, the bandages are taken off and a compression garment is fitted. If there is continuing reduction in limb circumference the treatment can be continued a third week. Any trunk oedema must be cleared first with massage.

The principles of bandaging are:

- Apply moisturizing cream to limb
- Cotton sleeve (Tubifast, red or yellow size)
- Bandage fingers (K-flex bandage)
- Pad creases with cotton wool
- Make limb into a cylinder (Velband or Dalzofoam)
- Apply low stretch bandage (Secure forte)
- Stockinette sleeve (stops bandage catching)

Before applying the bandages, the limb must be made into a cylinder using Velband (Johnson and Johnson) or Dalzofoam (Seton). The reason is that the pressure exerted by a bandage increases as the limb diameter decreases (Laplace's law), so an even limb diameter is needed to avoid areas of constriction.

Finger bandaging, using narrow gauge 2.5cm J Fast bandage (Johnson and Johnson) is done twice from tip to web; this is close-weave bandage (so that fluid does not push through). Crossovers, from each finger to wrist, go at the back of the hand (leaving the palm free).

Low stretch bandages are required for the arm or leg (not the high compression type used for venous ulcers). Secure forte (Johnson and Johnson) 8 or 10cm is a useful low stretch bandage. Scholl Poroplast 7.5cm is also good, and is slightly adhesive which make it easier to apply.

Start at the wrist or ankle with figures of 8 and spiral up the limb, covering half the bandage with each turn, reducing to a third as you near the axilla or groin. Secure the ends of the bandage with tape, not metal clips. A severly swollen limb may need a second bandage in figures of 8 up the limb. The patient should be able to move all joints after bandaging, and should be instructed to remove the bandaging if it becomes uncomfortably tight at any time. Each bandage lasts a day, but can sometimes be re-used to last 2 days.

Paroven may occasionally have a place in treating lymphoedema. It is licensed as a capilliary sealant for chronic venous insufficiency (oedema, cramps, restless legs), but there is no evidence that it is effective. However, in a double-blind cross-over trial in patients with lymphoedema of the arm or leg, Paroven 1g TDS for 6 months made the limbs become softer and symptoms were reduced. (Piller NB, *et al*, Br J Plast Surg 1988;78:1269-70)

A booklet that is very useful for patients and carers is "Lymphoedema-Advice on Treatment" by C Regnard, C Badger and P Mortimer (1988 and 1991). Beaconfields Publishers LTD.

LYMPHOMAS

Hodgkin's disease is the commonest malignancy of young adults. It usually presents with painless enlargement of nodes, but can spread to involve extra-nodal sites: lung, bowel, CNS, liver, bone marrow, skin, pharynx or eye. There is a good chance of cure at all stages, and even with advanced disease 40% survive 10 years.

Non-Hodgkin's lymphoma tends to present with more advanced disease, and diagnosis can be difficult if it presents at an extra-nodal site. High-grade lymphomas usually have histiocytic or undifferentiated histology. 40% can be cured with chemotherapy, but if there is no response death can occur within months. Low grade lymphomas (usually follicular histology) have a median survival of 8 years.

Problems in advanced lymphoma include:

- Node masses (respond to radiotherapy)
- Anaemia
- Bleeding (thrombocyopenia)
- Infections (thrush, herpes)
- CNS disease
- Sweats, itch, fever
- Spinal cord compression

MELANOMA

Melanoma causes about 1200 deaths per year in the UK. It is a rare skin tumour that presents as a mole that itches, bleeds, ulcerates or darkens. It should be general knowledge that such moles should be reported immediately. It is curable if excised at a very early stage (less than 0.75mm deep it has a 90% cure rate). Deeper tumours are widely excised and may require skin grafting. It can also originate in the eye, requiring enucleation.

Recurrent melanoma can occur many years after surgery or enucleation. Lymphatic recurrence is treated by block dissection or radiotherapy, but only 10% survive 5 years.

Metastases from melanoma occur to liver, bone, brain, spinal cord, skin and meninges (causing cranial nerve palsies and diplopia). Metastases are often rapidly growing and median survival is only 5 months. Although the primay tumours tend to be radio-resistant the metastases behave differently and will often respond to doses around 20-40 Gy, depending on the site.

Chemotherapy for melanoma with combinations of such drugs as procarbazine, vincristine, cisplatin, or lomustine, only produces a response in 20%, which may prolong life for 3-6 months. The response is usually confined to skin and lung metastases, No routine role for chemotherapy has been establised. Arterial limb perfusion with cytotoxics can occasionally be of help.

MENINGEAL METASTASES

Meningeal metastases (also called carcinomatous meningitis or carcinomatous infiltration of the meninges) occurs occasionally in lymphomas and leukaemias, but is rare in solid tumours. It occurs occasionally in breast cancer, small cell cancer of the lung and melanoma. Prognosis is usually very poor (1-2 months).

The clinical picture is typically one of neurological damage at several levels, with cranial nerve lesions (double vision, facial numbness, dysarthria) together with spinal cord involvement, and cortical effects due to restricted blood flow to the surface of the cerebral cortex. Symptoms include:

- headaches (neck stiffness may occur)
- cranial nerve lesions
- weak legs (back pain may occur)
- mental changes (mood, concentration)
- siezures (rarely)
- hydrocephalus

Diagnosis is usually clinical. MRI scan shows thickened meninges. CT scan may be normal or may show some hydrocephalus. A myelogram may show nodules on nerve root. CSF may contain malignant cells.

Treatment may be attempted with RT or intrathecal chemotherapy in relatively fit patients, in order to try to prevent progression to distressing neurological disability.

MESOTHELIOMA

Mesothelioma is a sarcomatous or anaplastic pleural tumour, caused by exposure to asbestosis in 90% of cases. Asbestos causes mesothelioma in 5-10% of people exposed to it, after 10-50 years. The association with asbestos was first described in 1960. It presents with chest pain or dyspnoea. Diagnosis may be suspected from CT scan which may show pleural thickening, and is confirmed by pleural biopsy, but the histology is often equivocal, and open thoracotomy is sometimes needed to make the diagnosis.

Treatment is very unsatisfactory. Surgery is attempted for localized tumours but recurrence is common. Radiotherapy and chemotherapy are tried but have little effect. Spread is local to the chest wall, and occasionally through the diaphragm to the peritoneal cavity, abdominal nodes and liver. It rarely involves the contra-lateral chest and rarely causes distant metastases.

Problems in advanced mesothelioma include:

- Pleural effusion
- Pain
- Chest infection

Pleural effusions can be tapped, but often become loculated eventually. Tumour nodules often develop at the site of needle puncture.

Pain may not respond completely to morphine and may require chest wall nerve blocks.

Chest infections tend to be recurrent and develop due to restricted lung expansion. Antibiotics are needed for symptoms.

METASTASES

A tumour starts as a single cell , and increases to reach 2,000,000,000 cells (about 2g in weight) before clinical effects begin to occur. Microscopic infiltration of blood and lymphatics usually occurs before the primary tumour becomes apparent. 2kg of tumour load (a further 1000 fold increase in size) is the maximum that the body can tolerate.

The organs affected by metastases (in order of frequency) are:

- Abdominal nodes
- Liver
- Lung
- Mediastinal nodes

- Pleura
- Bone
- Adrenal glands
- Peritoneum
- Brain
- Dura
- Pancreas
- Ovary
- Skin

(Information based on 1000 autopsies of cancer patients, Abrams, 1950). For some reason metastases never occur to heart, spleen or skeletal muscles, even though these organs have a rich blood supply. Small metastases may remain undetectable in life (especially in deep nodes, kidney or brain). Clinicians tend to underestimate the extent of metastases discovered at post-mortem.

The tendency to metastasize is very variable. Some tumours such as astrocytomas rarely cause metastases, whereas others such as small cell lung cancer, melanoma and testicular teratoma metastasize widely. The timing of metastases also varies, in that some tumours present with metastatic disease before the primary tumour is apparent (*see Unknown primary tumours*) whereas others may not develop metastases until years after the primary is treated, such as breast, kidney or melanoma. Spontaneous regression of metastases is well documented but exceedingly rare.

Lymph node involvement commonly occurs as a tumour spreads locally, and the spread usually occurs in a predictable anatomical order. Most malignant tumours spread to lymph nodes (although it is rare with sarcomas). Nodes replaced by tumour are usually enlarged. Superficial nodes in the neck, axillae and groins may ulcerate through the skin, when local RT can result in regression and sometimes healing.

Liver metastases occur in 40% of cancers. They are common with intra-abdominal malignancies, particularly stomach, pancreas, colon and rectum, because the portal venous system drains blood from these organs to the liver. Blood-borne spread also occurs from lung, breast and melanoma. Massive hepatomegaly can occur in melanoma. Liver function is often maintained and even with massive liver metastases liver failure is rare. Jaundice may be due to intra-hepatic metastases or external biliary compression. Liver metastases are usually multiple, when prognosis is only around 3 months from the time symptoms occur, but solitary metastases occur occasionally, when the prognosis from symptoms is around 18 months, and these may be resectable (*see Colon cancer*).

Lung metastases are seen in about 30% of patients with advanced cancer. They are particularly associated with renal cancers, sarcomas, testicular teratomas and osteosarcomas, but do also occur with the commoner cancers of breast prostate and colon. Pulmonary metastases at the pleural surface may cause a pleural effusion. Invasion of the chest wall may occur causing pain which may be controlled by RT. Large metastases tend to become haemorrhagic. Small lung metastases often cause little or no dyspnoea but extensive lung replacement will cause dsypnoea, which may be reduced by high dose steroids (*see dyspnoea*). Lung metastases are usually multiple, but solitary metastases occur (in renal cancers especially) and if there is no evidence of disease elsewhere on CT scan resection results in about 20% 5 year survival.

Bone metastases occur in about 25% of cancer patients. They are usually blood-borne, although direct invasion of bone can occur, especially in cancers of the head and neck and pelvis. Tumours that commonly cause bone metastases are breast, bronchus, prostate, kidney and thyroid. Prognosis with bone metastases from cancers of breast, prostate and myeloma can still be several years. The axial skeleton (containing red marrow) is the part that is affected: vertebrae, skull, pelvis, ribs, sternum, upper femur, upper humerus. Most metastases are predominantly osteolytic. Tumour cells cause bone damage by increasing the bone-resorbing activity of the osteoclasts (*see Bone pain*).

Brain metastases occur in 5-10% of cancer patients and are seen most commonly in cancers of breast, bronchus, gastro-intestinal tract, genito-urinary tract and melanoma. 80% occur in the cerebral hemispheres. (*see Brain Metastases*). Meningeal infiltration is associated with relapsing acute leukaemia but can occur rarely in solid tumours (*see Meningeal metastases*).

Body cavity metastases tend to be multiple serosal deposits and tend to cause effusions. Repeated paracentesis may cause fibrosis and loculation. Pleural and pericardial effusions are particularly associated with cancers of the breast, lung and oesophagus. Peritoneal metastases are particularly associated with cancers of the ovary and also colon, stomach and pancreas. (*see Ascites, Pleural effusion*)

Further Reading:
Carter RL. Some pathological aspects of advanced malignant disease, in Saunders C Ed, The management of terminal malignant disease, second edition, 1984, Edward Arnold.

MORPHINE

Morphine is an analgesic that acts as an agonist at the mu receptors in the brain and spinal cord. It is a naturally occuring alkaloid in the opium poppy (like codeine and papaveretum) but its chemical structure was elucidated in 1925, and it is now synthesised chemically.

Morphine is the drug of choice for continuous cancer pain (visceral or soft tissue pain). It is much less effective for intermittent pains (bone, nerve, colicy pains) when other approaches are needed (*see Pain*). A knowledge of morphine pharmacokinetics is <u>not</u> necessary in order to use the drug effectively.

Clinical principles of using morphine:

- Use for continuous pain
- 4 hourly dose
- Low dose initially
- Increase dose regularly
- 90% need 5-60mg 4 hourly
- Start a laxative day 1
- Be prepared to reduce the dose later

Use 4 hourly oral morphine initially, and start with a low dose, 2.5-5mg 4 hourly. If the patient is getting pain despite 4 hourly co-proxamol, then 10mg 4 hourly is usually needed. Increase the dose frequently, every 4 hours, (5, 10, 20, 30, 40, 60, 90mg morphine 4 hourly) until the patient is pain free for the entire 4 hour period. 90% of patients are pain-controlled on 5-60mg, but 10% require higher doses (and 1% of patients need very high doses above 500mg 4 hourly). Once the correct dose is established and the patient is pain-free for the full 4 hours, then 12 hourly MST can be used as an alternative.

Note: If fluid retention, ascites or pleural effusion develop the dose may need to be increased, because the morphine is distributed in a larger volume of body fluid.

5 Clinical rules when using morphine:

1.   If any opioid drug reduces the pain a bit, it is usually possible to achieve total pain control with the correct dose.
2.   The rule for increasing the dose is "If the morphine is helping and the patient is not drowsy, increase the dose". Once the correct dose is established and the patient is pain-free for the full 4 hours, then 12 hourly MST can be used as an alternative.
3.   When increasing the dose, increase by about 50% (even at high doses). For example, a patient on oral morphine 30mg 4 hourly who had pain breakthrough after 3 hours could be increased to oral morphine 45mg 4 hourly. A patient on MST 400mg BD who developed pain breakthrough after 10-11 hours could be increased to MST 600mg BD.
4.   The rule for decreasing the dose is: "Pain-free and drowsy, reduce the dose". The longer a patient is on morphine the more likely they are to need a reduction in dose, because pain fluctuates. Ask regularly about drowsiness.
5.   After a nerve blocking procedure (and sometimes after radiotherapy or chemotherapy) pain may be reduced or abolished, and the morphine dose should then be reduced and re-titrated from 5mg 4 hourly as an inpatient, to avoid excessive drowsiness or even respiratory depression.

Various forms of morphine are available including:

- Aqueous morphine (in chloroform water)
- Oramorph solution (10mg in 5ml)
- Oramorph solution (100mg in 5ml)
- Sevredol tablets (10mg blue, 20mg pink)
- Slow-release 12 hourly morphine (MST, SRM-retard)

4 hourly morphine (Oramorph solution or Sevredol tablets) should be used initially, starting with a low dose, 2.5-5mg 4 hourly. Once a steady dose is achieved, transfer to slow release morphine. Sevredol tablets are useful for controlling breakthrough pain in a patient on 12 hourly MST.

Morphine suppositories usually 10mg and 30mg (but can be higher doses can be made up) are effective, but only for 4 hours. If a suppository regime is needed then oxycodone suppositories, which last 8 hours, are preferable (see Analgesics).

Mixed opium alkaloids (nepenthe and papaveretum) should be avoided. They contain morphine and other alkaloids and have no advantages over pure morphine. Avoid morphine combinations such as Cyclimorph (cyclizine plus morphine) or combination elixirs which can cause excessive drowsiness.

Slow-release morphine (MST, SRM-Rhotard) is very helpful and effective. 12 hourly medication eases the burden of tablet-taking. The ideal method is to start 4 hourly morphine and transfer to a slow-release preparation when the patient's requirement is established. The following strengths are available:

SLOW RELEASE MORPHINE TABLETS		
10mg	–	yellow
15mg	–	green
30mg	–	purple
60mg	–	orange
100mg	–	grey
200mg		blue

If starting on MST, the starting dose is 10-30mg BD. If a patient has not been on morphine before, it is often sensible to start with 10-20mg BD with the option of increasing the dose as needed, because starting at 30mg BD may cause drowsiness which puts the patient off using it.

Slow-release morphine is designed for 12 hourly release. If pain breakthrough occurs, increase the 12 hourly dose. A very small number of patients seem to experience pain breakthrough after 10-11 hours, whatever the dose, and a TID regime is then more suitable.

Before a nerve blocking procedure, MST should be stopped and 4 hourly morphine should be re-started, so that if pain is abolished the dose of morphine can be stopped quickly.

Absorbtion of MST is delayed by paralytic ileus and therefore MST should not be used for post-operative pain, when sequestered tablets may suddenly get absorbed as bowel function returns, causing overdose. Absorbtion is also reduced by a fatty meal and probably in some cases of intestinal obstruction.

Rectal MST is equally effective as oral MST. Although not licensed for rectal use, the oral tablets can be given rectally, and this is occasionally very useful in the home care situation. In one study, 38 patients with advanced cancer who had been pain-controlled on oral MST, were transferred to the same dose of rectal MST (dose range 60-300mg 12 hourly) because of nausea or dysphagia. Pain control was maintained in all cases. In 11 patients the rectal dose needed to be reduced because of drowsiness, suggesting even better absortion than the oral route. The duration of rectal use ranged from 1-30 days. No rectal soreness occured (Reference: Maloney CM *et al.* The rectal administration of MS-Contin: clinical implications of use in end stage cancer. The American Journal of Hospice Care July\August 1989: 34-35).

Diamorphine injections are used, rather than morphine injections, because of diamorphine's high solubility. Diamorphine is simply a pro-drug of morphine, and rapidly converted to morphine in the body. 400mg diamorphine will dissolve in 1ml of water, whereas it would take 10ml of water to dissolve 400mg morphine. The injected dose of diamorphine is 50% of the oral dose of morphine (*see Diamorphine*).

Nebulized morphine has been used to control pain quickly at the site of accidents, and in the treatment of chronic dyspnoea. Morphine is poorly absorbed by the inhaled route (10% absorbtion) but may act at opiod receptors in the lung to reduce dyspnoea. The pharmacokinetics of its absorbtion by this route requires further study (*see Dyspnoea*).

Side-effects of morphine include:

- Constipation
- Nausea or vomiting (30% for 48 hours)
- Drowsiness (dose too high)
- Respiratory depression (in massive overdose)
- Dry mouth
- Sweating (rare)
- Itch (20% after spinal morphine)
- Constriction of the pupils
- Bronchoconstriction (mild)
- Increased biliary tone

The last 3 side-effects occur because morphine is an agonist at opioid receptors in the iris, gut and bronchial epithelium, as well as the CNS.

Drug interactions with morphine are rare, the most important one being with MAOI anti-depressants, when hypertensive crisis and mental agitation can occur.

Alcohol is safe for patients on morphine, even very high dose morphine, with no adverse effects. Most hospices have a drinks trolley that precedes the evening drugs trolley on its rounds (*see Alcohol*).

The morphine myths include:

- Respiratory depression
- Addiction
- Tolerance
- Euphoria

Respiratory depression is preceded by drowsiness. This does not occur if the dose is reduced whenever a patient on morphine becomes painfree and drowsy. Pain prevents respiratory depression by stimulating the respiratory centre. Animal studies have demonstrated pain fibres connecting with the medullary respiratory centre. If pain is abolished (e.g. with a nerve block) then morphine can rapidly cause respiratory depression.

Addiction is feared by many patients, (even though it is less relevant if their life is short anyway). But in fact it cannot occur if a patient has morphine-responsive pain. This is well demonstrated by patients on high doses of morphine, who have an effective nerve block and stop morphine immediately, with no ill effects. This could not happen in a patient without pain, who would experience very unpleasant physical and psychological effects of suddenly stopping a high regular dose.

Tolerance (needing higher and higher doses with diminishing analgesic effect) is also feared by patients ("If I start it now, it won't work when the pain gets really bad"). In fact tolerance does not occur when morphine is used for continuous cancer pain. Many patients stay on the same dose for weeks or months and many patients need to reduce the dose at some stage. The myth of tolerance has arisen because if morphine is given for some pains (bone, nerve) it does not abolish the pain, but because the patient has pain they can tolerate morphine without drowsiness. Since they still have pain, the dose is increased and increased, usually to no effect. It is essential to assess the pain before starting morphine (see Pain).

Euphoria is another myth. Morphine used as a regular analgesic has no direct effect on mood. Any improvement in mood is due to pain relief. There is some evidence that high doses long-term may contribute to depression.

Stopping longterm morphine is occasionally necessary, in a patient who no longer has pain but has become accustomed to the morphine. Morphine used with pain cannot become addictive, but longterm morphine without pain can. The dose can be reduced gradually every day, and when it is finally stopped methadone linctus (2mg\5ml) should be given TID for a few days and gradually reduced, to prevent symptoms of withdrawal.

Children with continuous pain or severe dyspnoea benefit from morphine in the same way as adults. In a survey of 50 children, aged 1-14, in a hospice, 50% needed less than 20mg 4 hourly, but some needed high doses up to 360mg 4 hourly. Respiratory depression was not seen. (Palliative Medicine 1987; 1: 27-30).

Morphine overdose is extremely rare in hospice practice, but may occur from a prescribing error, or as a deliberate overdose or following a nerve block. Accidental overdose is usually safe in patients established on morphine, when a single dose 5-10 times the routine dose is only likely to cause drowsiness for a few hours (Reference: O'Neill WM. Safety of Diamorphine in overdose. Palliative Medicine 1989; 3: 307-309). The signs of significant overdose are:
  • Coma

- Slow respirations (around 5 per minute)
- Pinpoint pupils

Naloxone reverses the effects of morphine, but must be used very carefully, otherwise the patient may experience severe pain breakthrough and severe withdrawal phenomena (sweats, tachycardia, twitching, panic). 0.1mg IV will be enough to improve respirations, but the effect is short-lived and it may need to be repeated every 15-60 minutes.

Travelling abroad with morphine may require an export licence, if travelling for longer than 15 days or taking more than 1.2g of morphine. It is sensible to also discuss local regulations with the embassy concerned. The licence is easily obtained (allow 10 days) by sending a supporting letter from a doctor (drug details, travel dates) to:

> Home Office
> Drugs Branch
> Queen Anne's Gate
> London SW1H 9AT
> Tel. 071 213 5357

Driving is possible, and legal, when a patient is established on a steady dose of morphine that is controlling pain without causing any drowsiness.

Prescribing morphine and other controlled drugs involves following certain legal requirements (Misuse of Drugs Regulations, 1985). It is an offence to issue an incomplete prescription. The requirements are:

- Prescriber's own handwriting
- Prescriber's address stamped on
- Name and address of patient
- Form and strength of preparation
- Total quantity in words and figures
- Dose prescribed
- Signed and dated by prescriber

The pharmacology of morphine has been poorly understood until recently, partly because of the difficulty in developing accurate assays to measure morphine and its metabolites in body tissues. There is no correlation between plasma levels and analgesic effect. Even with a constant dose in a single patient the plasma level varies.

Absorbtion of morphine is 100% by the small bowel. It is also well absorbed by the buccal and rectal mucosa, (which can be useful in some clinical situations, e.g. aqueous morphine trickled into the mouth of a dying patient is well absorbed, and rectal MST is well absorbed, so that if for some reason the patient is unable to swallow their MST tablets they are just as effective if they are given rectally).

Liver metabolism means that there is little morphine left (only about 30% of the oral dose) to reach the circulation, and this poor oral bioavailability was difficult to understand in a drug that was so effective. This is now explained by the fact that its metabolite, morphine 6 glucuronide (M6G) is also powerfully analgesic, acting at the mu receptors, and in repeated doses the level of M6G builds up in the CSF, explaining why repeated doses of morphine are much more effective than a single dose.

M6G is an analgesic in its own right. M6G has been given to man and is about 3-4 times as potent as morphine. Other metabolites, M3G and normorphine, do not cross the blood brain barrier and are not active as metabolites.

Opioid receptors were postulated in 1954 to explain the dual action of nalorphine, an analgesic which nevertheless antagonizes morphine. This is now explained in terms of its agonist\antagonist properties, agonist at the kappa receptors, but antagonist at the mu receptors, where morphine acts. In 1969 endogenous opioids were postulated, by Reynolds, an experimental psychologist, to explain the observation that midbrain stimulation in rats produced total-body analgesia. The midbrain is rich in opioid receptors and inhibitory fibres have since been identified that pass from the midbrain to the dorsal horn of the spinal cord. By 1973 opioid receptors had been identified as present in all vertebrates, making it clear that it is a very primitive analgesic system in the body. In 1975 Kosterlitz and Hughes identified endogenous opioids (from pigs brains) and found that they displaced morphine from opioid receptors.

Further reading:
Hanks GW, Hoskins PJ, Opioid analgesics in the management of pain in patients with cancer. A review. Palliative Medicine 1987; 1: 1-25.
Gorman DJ Opioid analgesia in the management of pain in patients with cancer: an update. Palliative Medicine 1991; 5: 277-294

MOTOR NEURONE DISEASE

Motor Neurone Disease (MND) is a disease characterized by the degeneration of motor nerves. It causes progressive weakness, dependency and death. It was first described in 1850. The cause remains unknown. It is rare, affecting 5 per 100,000 of the population. The peak age is 60-80, but it can occur in young adults. It is slightly more common in men (3:2). The nerve cells affected are:

- Anterior horn cells (wasting)
- Cortico-spinal tracts (spasticity)
- Brain stem (bulbar palsy)

A patient with MND wrote: "Doctors of today should not feel that because they cannot cure patients with Motor Neurone Disease they cannot help them. They can indeed help them by their compassionate understanding and friendship". A review of 100 patients with MND at St Christopher's Hospice emphasized what a difference a determined programme of symptom control and psychological support can make.

Presentation of MND is with weakness or clumsiness of an arm or leg, or slurring of words. Diagnosis is often delayed. Median time from presentation to diagnosis is 13 months.

Median survival in MND is 2-3 years from diagnosis. 20% survive 5 years, 10% survive 10 years. Survival tends to be shorter in the elderly and with bulbar symptoms. Poor basal expansion on inspiration is a sign of a short prognosis.

Diagnosis of MND is clinical and based on a combination of:

- Fasciculations (muscle twitches)
- Wasting
- Spasticity

Fasciculations of the muscles of the arms and tongue together with spasticity in the legs is diagnostic. The main differential diagnosis is cord compression due to cervical spondylosis, which can also cause flaccid weakness in the arms, sometimes with local fasciculations, due to nerve root damage (but without the widespread fasciculations) and spastic weakness in the legs. A myelogram may be indicated to exclude cervical cord damage. Electromyography confirms the diagnosis of MND by showing fibrillations at rest and reduced spikes (of poor amplitude) with contractions.

Symptoms of motor neurone disease include:

- Weakness
- Speech problems
- Tiredness (lack of energy)
- Muscle spasms (*see Muscle spasms*)
- Pain (aching joints, skin pressure)
- Dyspnoea
- Dsyphagia
- Emotional lability (uncontrollable laughing\crying)
- Dribbling
- Sore eyes from reduced blinking (hypromellose drops)

Attention to detail is the key. What is helpful to one patient can be unbearable to another.

Immobility is the big problem in MND. "When a person is paralysed quite ordinary discomforts assume the character of minor tortures". Immobility can cause the following problems:

- Constipation
- Urinary retention
- Pressure sores
- Anxiety, depression
- Panic
- Insomnia
- Boredom

A sensitive switch is essential when nursing a patient with advanced MND. "It is not realized that fear amounting to panic occurs by day or night, and it is therefore essential that help should be available. Contact can be made by means of a bell or buzzer which responds to the slightest touch".

What is not affected by MND? It can be reassuring to know that this progressive disease leaves some parts of the body unaffected. Many people confuse MND with multiple sclerosis. MND does not affect:

- Sensation
- Vision, eye movements
- Hearing
- Brain function
- Smooth muscles (heart)
- Bladder or bowel muscle
- Sexual function

N.B. MND is rarely hereditary. A familial (dominantly inherited) form occurs in about 5% of patients.

All patients with MND should be offered:

- A key-worker
- Regular symptom control
- Physiotherapy
- O.T.
- S.W. – finances, employment, housing
- Family counselling
- Respite admissions
- Contact with MND association

Equipment must be ordered skillfully as the disease progresses. An experienced OT should always be consulted. Consider referral to a specialized unit for assessment, such as Mary Marlborough Lodge, Nuffield Orthopaedic Centre, Oxford, Tel. 0865 64811. The aim is to avoid the patient and family saying: "if only we had had this 2 months ago". There is a vast array of useful aids and equipment to help with:

- Mobility
- Driving
- Sitting
- Transfers
- Positioning
- Skin care
- Eating
- Bathing
- Toileting
- Reading
- Communicating
- Controlling the environment (POSSUM)

Communication aids are developing all the time, and a thorough assessment at a communication aids centre is essential before buying expensive equipment. Simple equipment is sometimes all that is needed. Consider:

- Alphabet chart or picture chart
- Eye-pointing chart (E-tran board)
- Cannon communicator
- Lightwriter
- Lap-top computer with appropriate software
- POSSUM – patient-operated environmental control system including a communication facility.

POSSUM can control many aspects of the patient's environment from a single switch. Address: Possum Controls LTD, Middlegreen Rd, Langley, Slough, Berkshire, SL3 6DF Tel. 0753 579234.

Counselling in MND is especially important at crisis points of deterioration and change. Feelings of uncertainty and abandonment are the greatest sources of despair. "Being told the disease was a progressive one enabled me to do things while I could". Explanation and reasurance of future support greatly raise morale. "With the practical help and prayers of others I have found it possible to set aside the physical and let the mental and spiritual take over. This is a very enriching experience". Isolation is a common feeling. "Loneliness is not so much a matter of being alone as of not belonging". Many patients with MND have never heard of the disease or anyone with it. The patient should be encouraged to join the MND association. Articles written by patients with MND can be very helpful. Two such articles are: Henke E. Motor neurone disease – a patient's view. BMJ 1968; 2:765 and Pollard D. Personal View. BMJ, 1984; 288: 481.

Dysphagia is common, but most patients can continue to feed orally with routine care. The following can be helpful:

- Neck positioning
- Speech therapist's assessment
- Ice
- Palatal plate
- Myotomy
- NG feeding
- Gastrostomy (*see Dysphagia*)

Careful positioning of the neck while eating is often the key to improved swallowing. It is very difficult to swallow if the neck is either too flexed or too extended. (Try it!). A speech therapist can analyse which part of the swallowing sequence has been affected: lip closure, tongue movement or bolus formation. Firm lip closure is the first part of normal swallowing. The tongue and mouth normally press a firm bolus of food onto the back of the pharynx which initiates the pharngeal reflex phase of swallowing. Getting food to the back of the mouth may be impossible with a weak tongue, and carers may need to place food at the back of the mouth. Semi-solid food forms a better bolus than liquids, and is therefore easier to swallow. Ice can improve the swallowing reflex by reducing muscle spasm. Sucking ice chips before a meal or holding a bag of frozen peas against the front of the neck for a few minutes before starting to eat, can improve swallowing. A palatal plate can help to prevent nasal regurgitation. It is a plastic extension to an existing denture or removable plate. It helps to close the soft palate during swallowing. Crico-pharyngeal myotomy is only helpful if there is pharyngeal spasm – best seen on cine radiography of a barium swallow. The patient complains of an obstruction in the throat and may get episodes of choking after eating due to aspiration of pooled food. Nasogastric tube feeding may be indicated if a patient is becoming exhausted by meals or is troubled by repeated choking. A fine bore tube can be well tolerated for a few days. Intermittent feeding for 24-48 hours every few days can keep the patient hydrated. Some patients want to go on eating despite all the difficulties to maintain normality. On the other hand some patients find it a relief to give up the daily battle with food. Percutaneous endoscopic gastrostomy is a simple technique which should be considered early on (see Dysphagia).

Dribbling is due to reduced swallowing. The following may help:

- Polo-neck bib to protect clothes
- Atropine (0.3mg 8hourly to 0.6mg 4 hourly)
- Palatal lift
- Portable suction (used carefully)
- Bilateral neurectomy to reduce salivation (rarely)

Choking is a cough reflex to protect the lungs and occurs if liquid is inhaled. It is worsened by panic. If recurrent, it is managed as dysphagia.

Morphine is useful in 85% at some stage. Morphine will control continuous pains (aching joints, skin pressure) and helps provide a good night's sleep if pain is causing insomnia. It can be safely given for months or years. Start with a low dose. Morphine is often helpful in the terminal phase to control dyspnoea (see Morphine).

Mode of death is usually due to respiratory failure, either gradual or sudden, and with medication is peaceful and settled in 95%. "The term choking is both inaccurate and inappropriate in describing the cause of death ... and its use should be abandoned" (O'Brien et al.). The MND association has produced a "Breathing Space" kit containing emergency drugs for the home, in the event of breathing difficulties.

The MND Association: 10 Notre Dame Mews, Albert Place, Northampton NN1 2BG, Telephone 0604-250505 offers:

- Information
- Leaflets – wide variety
- Equipment loans
- Newsletter
- Support for Research
- Helpline 0345-626262, Mon-Fri   9am-10-30pm

Further reading:
Cochrane GM, 1987, The Management of Motor Neurone Disease, Churchill Livingstone (104 pages).
O'Brien T, Kelly M, Saunders C, Motor neurone disease: a hospice perspective. BMJ 1992;304:471-3 (22 Feb 1992).

MOUTH PROBLEMS

Mouthcare is important. In a survey of hospice patients, 176 out of 197 patients (89%) had mouth problems (Jobbins *et al*, 1992), including:

- Thrush 85%
- Dry mouth 77%
- Denture problems 45%
- Taste disturbance 37%
- Oral soreness 33%

Oral thrush occurs in 85% of hospice patients on culture, but is not always symptomatic. It can cause dryness or soreness. Steroids and antibiotics predispose to thrush. Treat with nystatin or ketoconazole (*see Thrush*).

Routine mouthcare (2-4 hourly) is important for patient comfort, and involves

- Toothbrushing
- Mouthwash
- Cleansing with foamstick applicator
- Vaseline (thinly) to dry lips

Foamstick applicators are used after each meal so food is not lodged in the mouth. Crushed ice is soothing in the terminal stages.

Mouthwashes are mild antiseptics and are refreshing and prevent gingivitis. Mouthwashes for routine care include:

- 0.1% hexitidine (Oraldene)
- Thymol glycerin solution
- Effervescent mouthwash tablet
- 6% hydrogen peroxide – to remove debris
- 1% povidone iodine (Betadine) – for oral infection

Dry mouth may be due to drugs, dehydration or thrush. Many drugs can cause a dry mouth (morphine, anti-cholinergics, phenothiazines, diuretics). Dehydration causes a dry mouth, which is best managed with regular mouth care rather than IV fluids.

Glandosane spray (artificial saliva), ordinary or lemon flavour, used PRN, can be helpful for a dry mouth, that does not respond to other measures.

Denture problems are common. Wasting of the facial muscles causes looseness of the plate. This causes difficulty eating and embarrassment as the denture keeps falling down. It is a simple matter for the dentist to reline dentures so that they fit properly (and this is often a big boost to morale). Dentures should be removed at night and soaked in dental cleanser.

Taste disturbances are common, and occur in about 20% of hospice patients. Favourite tastes may suddenly become unpleasant. Food may taste too sweet or too salty. It can occur after certain cytotoxics (especially cytarabine). Adding herbs and spices to cooking sometimes helps. Taste changes are not necessarily permanent and after several weeks taste can return to normal. A bad taste in the mouth may be due to gingivitis, bleeding or thrush.

Soreness of the mouth may be due to:

- Thrush
- Loose dentures
- Mouth ulcers
- Radiation stomatitis
- Gingivitis

Benzydamine (Difflam), rinse or spray, is described as an oral analgesic, and gives 1-2 hours of partial numbness. An alternative is 2% lignocaine viscous mouthwash. Gingivitis is unusual, perhaps because of altered immuniity. Treat with metronidazole and Betadine mouthwash.

Coated tongue is unpleasant (and may be a startling black colour due to "black hairy tongue" which is a harmless fungal growth). Treatment can be with:

- Bocasan mouthwash
- Effervescent vitamin C
- Fresh pineapple
- Hydrogen peroxide mouthwash
- Miconazole gel on the tongue

Bocasan mouthwash (Oral-B) contains sodium perborate and helps clean a coated tongue. It is used 3 times a day. It must not be swallowed. Effervescent Vitamin C tablet (usually half a tablet) placed on the tongue daily or BD, can effectively remove any coating on the tongue. Fresh pineapple contains ananase, a proteolytic enzyme, and is best used in thin slices, frozen and coated in icing sugar (to prevent stinging). Hydrogen peroxide clears debris, but is unpleasant to use. Miconazole (Daktarin) gel applied to the tongue and removed with a soft brush will remove a black coating.

Mouth ulcers can be soothed using

- Choline salycilate gel (Bonjela)
- Triamcinolone paste (Adcortyl in orabase)
- 2.5% hydrocortisone pellets (Corlan)
- Benzocaine (Dequacaine) lozenges (short-acting)

Herpetic ulceration in AIDS is treated (or prevented) with oral acyclovir (Zovirax) 400mg 5 times a day, plus locally applied cream. Thalidomide 100mg BD has been reported as successful in healing idiopathic apthous ulcers (Ruvuz *et al.* 1990) and AIDS-associated oesophageal ulceration (New England Journal of Medicine, 16 July 1992, pp. 208–9). The mechanism of action is unknown. Long-term usage may cause a sensory neuropathy.

Reference:
Regnard C, Fitton S. Mouth Care: a flow diagram. Palliative Medicine 1989; 3: 67-69.
Jobbins J *et al.* Oral and dental disease in terminally ill cancer patients. Br Med J 1992; 304: 1612.
Ruvuz J *et al.* Crossover study of thalidomide vs placebo in severe recurrent apthous stomatitis. Arch Dermatol 1990; 126: 923-7.

MUSCLE SPASMS

Painful muscle spasms occur in MND and in spastic paraplegia due to cord damage. The dose of medication to control spasms needs to be balanced so that the spasms are reduced without causing floppiness, particularly of the trunk muscles.

Baclofen (Lioresal), 5-30mg TID, acts at the spinal level to reduce spasm. It should be taken after food to avoid nausea. It can cause confusion. Baclofen and Dantrolene can be used together.

Dantrolene (Dantrium), 25-100mg TID, acts directly on muscle to reduce spasm. Increase the dose gradually for full effect, which may take 6 weeks. Check LFTs after 6 weeks.

Diazepam (Valium) 2-10mg at night, can be useful for night spasms.

Quinine sulphate, 125mg, 200mg or 300mg at night can reduce night cramps. side-effects include headache, tinnitus and nausea.

MYELOMA

Myeloma causes about 2400 deaths per year in the UK. It is a malignancy of the plasma cells and occurs most commonly between 50-70 years. It is characterized by:

- Abnormal serum proteins
- Abnormal urinary proteins (Bence Jones proteins)
- Bone pains
- Anaemia
- Renal damage
- Hypercalcaemia (30%)

Diagnosis of myeloma is suspected if the ESR is above 100 and confirmed by detecting abnormal proteins (excessive immunoglobulins) by plasma electrophoresis. The bone lesions are entirely osteolytic and not detectable on bone scan.

Plasmacytoma is a solitary deposit of myeloma tissue (usually in bone or soft tissue) that can sometimes be cured with radiotherapy. Some cases progress to myeloma.

Chemotherapy for myeloma with melphalan and prednisolone improves prognosis from an average of 6-12 to 24-36 months. Radiotherapy is given for bone pains and dialysis is considered for renal failure.

Problems in advanced myeloma involves:

- Bone pains
- Vertebral collapse
- Cord compression (15%)
- Anaemia
- Infections
- Renal Failure
- Bleeding tendency (low platelets)
- Soft tissue lumps
- Hypercalcaemia

Hypercalcaemia occurs in 30% and may respond to steroids alone (unlike solid tumours). Soft tissue tumours shrink with radiotherapy. Death is usually due to a chest infection or uraemia.

NAUSEA AND VOMITING

Vomiting is the forceful expulsion of gastric contents. It is presumably a primitive mechanism intended to protect the body from ingesting harmful substances

Nausea is an unpleasant sensation that may precede vomiting, associated with salivation, sweating and tachycardia. Being invisible, it is more easily overlooked, and it is a more unpleasant symptom than vomiting alone, and is rated by patients as distressing as pain.

Incidence of nausea and vomiting is 50% of patients with advanced cancer (at some time) and 30% of patients on admission to a hospice. Most patients with nausea or vomiting can be managed at home.

The mechanism of nausea and vomiting is poorly understood (*see Anti-emetics*). The Chemo-receptor trigger zone, stimulated by drugs or chemicals (such as urea) is only one of many factors that act on the vomiting centre. Gastric stasis has been shown to occur in some cancer patients with intractable nausea and poor gastric emptying (Reference: Bruera *et al*, Journal of Pain and Symptom Control 1987; 2: 19-21). Other factors that can cause vomiting are:

- Sights, smells, taste
- Memories
- Motion
- Pharyngeal stimulation (cough)
- Gut receptors

The vomiting reflex is controlled by the vomiting centre which causes retching (diaphragmatic spasms against a closed glottis) with negative intra-thoracic pressure, so that food is drawn up into the oesophagus. Reverse peristalsis of the oesophagus then causes the vomiting. The vomiting reflex involves:

- Nausea (salivation, sweating, tachycardia)
- Gastric stasis
- Retching (diaphragmatic spasms) with
- Closure of the vocal cords
- Elevation of the palate (closing the nose)
- Reverse peristalsis of oesophagus

Assessment of nausea and vomiting involves taking a detailed history of the pattern of vomiting (speed of onset, pattern, precipitating factors) including previous anti-emetics tried, and in what doses. Ask about:

- Surgery to bowel?
- Drugs
- Reflux or hiccups?
- Dyspepsia?
- Thirst or drowsiness (hypercalcaemia)
- Constipation
- Dysuria

Vomiting with little nausea suggests:

- Gastric stasis (large volumes, reflux)
- Squashed stomach (small volumes, reflux)
- Gastric obstruction (large volumes, forceful)
- Raised ICP

Examine the patient for papilloedema and thrush and examine the abdomen including a PR, look for neurological signs and take blood (U and Es, calcium) and send an MSU.

Management of nausea and vomiting aims to control nausea and vomiting as quickly as possible. The first aim in treatment is to abolish nausea. Patients can tolerate occasional vomiting, provided they are free of nausea. 30% of patients require 2 anti-emetics (*see Anti-emetics*). Management involves the following steps:

- Exclude reversible causes
- Choose appropriate anti-emetic
- Choose route: PR or SC?
- Consider steroids

Reversible causes of nausea and vomiting (*see table*) are most commonly drug-induced, anxiety, constipation, heartburn, thrush or urinary infection. Drugs that cause nausea include morphine oestrogens, digoxin, antibiotics (especially erythromycin and metronidazole) iron, theophyllines and cytotoxics (*see Chemotherapy*). Susceptibility to motion sickness may predict the severity of chemotherapy-induced vomiting. Anxiety is a common factor and may be partially denied (hence it emerges as nausea). Anti-emetics alone are not usually enough to control it. Consider asking "Have you known anyone else with cancer?" or "What do you think this sickness may be caused by?" Hypercalcaemia due to myeloma may respond to steroids, but in solid tumours hypercalcaemia responds partially or poorly to steroids and other measures are needed. (*see Hypercalcaemia*).

REVERSIBLE CAUSES OF NAUSEA AND VOMITING

CAUSE	FEATURES	TREATMENT
Drugs	Recently started? Digoxin level?	Stop or reduce drug
Anxiety	"Sick with fear." Situational. Patient may not recognize anxiety. Anti-emetics are not effective	Anxiolytics Counselling
Brain metastases	Headaches Neurological signs Projectile vomits Little nausea	Steroids
Oral Thrush	White plaques	Ketoconazole
Gastric irritation	NSAIDs	Ranitidine Change NSAID?
Squashed Stomach Syndrome	Fullness Heartburn Nausea on eating	Antacids Ranitidine Metoclopramide
Gastric Outflow Obstruction	Large volume vomit every 1-2 days. Little nausea	Steroids
Constipation	History PR examination	Laxatives Enemas
Cough	Vomiting after bout of coughing. Little nausea	Antitussives Antibiotics Nebulizer

CAUSE	FEATURES	TREATMENT
UTI	Smelly urine Frequency, incontinence (or no features)	MSU Antibiotics
Hypercalcaemia	Drowsiness Thirst	Rehydrate Pamidronate
Uraemia	Hiccups Twitching	Explain to relatives

Anti-emetics are required when reversible causes are being treated, and for non-reversible causes, such as tumour load, liver metastases or intestinal obstruction. Anti-emetics that are particularly useful (*see also Anti-emetics*) are:

- Cyclizine
- Metoclopramide
- Haloperidol
- Methotrimeprazine

The route of anti-emetics is important. Oral anti-emetics are only effective in preventing nausea or treating mild nausea. For the control of nausea or vomiting, anti-emetics need to be given by suppository, injection or SC infusion, because nausea causes gastric stasis and prevents the absorbtion of oral drugs. Anti-emetic suppositories can be useful in the home to control mild nausea and vomiting before reverting to oral anti-emetics. The following are used:

- Prochlorperazine (Stemetil), 25mg 8 hourly
- Domperidone (Motilium), 30-60mg 6 hourly
- Cyclizine (Valoid), 50mg 6-8 hourly

Subcutaneous infusions of anti-emetics are particularly useful to gain control of nausea or vomiting or for the longterm management of malignant intestinal obstruction. Every GP practice should have its own syringe pump. (*see Subcutanous infusions*). The following drugs are commonly used:

	Usual starting dose per 24 hours
• Cyclizine	150mg
• Metoclopramide	40mg
• Haloperidol	5mg
• Methotrimeprazine	75mg

Dexamethasone can be added to a SC infusion and enhances the anti-emetic action of metoclopramide, and probably other anti-emetics as well. In severe nausea or vomiting that is not responding to anti-emetics, the addition of dexamethasone will often help. Steroids are also used to control nausea or vomiting in several specific situations:

- Raised intracranial pressure
- High obstruction
- Hypercalcaemia in myeloma
- Anti-emetic resistance

Persistent nausea or vomiting is unusual if the above measures are taken. Possible causes are:

- Conditioned response
- Anxiety
- High intestinal obstruction
- Brainstem metastasis (rare)

Conditioned responses from familiar smells and sights can become associated with severe nausea. A few days of high dose anti-emetics can break the cycle. The patient will usually tolerate some sedation if the aim of treatment is explained. After a few days free of nausea, the doses of anti-emetics can be gradually reduced.

Anxiety can occur as an effect of the vomiting ("Is the cancer spreading?"). There may also be social and emotional reasons for anxiety, which if severe may require hospice type admission to control.

High obstruction may occur at the pylorus or duodenum. There is a picture of forceful large-volume vomits of undigested food. A palliative gastro-enterostomy should be considered. Dexamethasone 8-12mg daily will relieve the vomiting in around 50% but may take several days to be effective. The patient may prefer a nasogastric tube to repeated vomiting. An alternative may be to use octreotide (see *Intestinal obstruction*).

Brain tumours in the floor of the fourth ventricle affecting the CTZ can cause intractable vomiting relieved by discrete surgical lesions (Reference: Lindstrom PA Brizzee KR, Relief of intractable vomiting from surgical lesions in area postrema, J Neurosurg 1962;19:228-36)

Treatment of persistent nausea or vomiting can be with a 24 hour subcutaneous infusion of cyclizine 150mg, plus metoclopramide 60mg, or methotrimeprazine 75-150mg. High dose methotrimeprazine will cause sedation, but this will usually be tolerated as preferable to severe nausea, and once the nausea settles, the dose can be gradually reduced. Dexamethasone 6-12mg per 24 hours has an additional anti-emetic action. If anxiety is playing a part, the addition of SC midazolam 20-60mg per 24 hours, can be very helpful.

Dietary advice in persistent nausea includes:

- Avoid strong cooking smells
- Small meals (2-3 spoonfuls)
- Try cold foods
- Try tonic water

Ondansetron may have a place in treating severe intractable nausea or vomiting, not responding to the above measures. IV ondansetron 8mg BD may be effective when other methods fail (Case report of 1 patient, Lancet 22 February 1992, p490). Ondansetron by SC infusion or orally may be especially useful to control intractable vomiting due to raised ICP. (Palliative Medicine 1992; 6; 167 – case report).

Coeliac plexus block is said to control intractable nausea, if all else fails (although I have never seen it needed).

References:
Allan SG. Review article: Emesis in the patient with advanced cancer. Palliative Medicine 1988; 2: 89-100.
Regnard C, Comiskey M. Nausea and vomiting in advanced cancer – a flow diagram. Palliative Medicine 1992; 6: 146-151.

NERVE BLOCKS

Nerve blocks are procedures to control localized pain by blocking nerve conduction (either temporarily or permanently). 7% of hospice patients benefit from a nerve block. The indication for a nerve block is pain that is not adequately controlled by other methods: morphine, NSAIDs, steroids other co-analgesics or radiotherapy. N.B. A nerve block can be worthwhile even if a patient only has a short prognosis. The most useful nerve blocks are:

NERVE BLOCK	PAIN
Coeliac Plexus	– Abdominal
Paravertebral	– Chest wall
Intercostal	– Rib
Brachial Plexus	– Arm
Steroid injection	– Rib\Vertebra
Hip	– Hip
Intrathecal	– Perineal
Lumbar Sympathetic	– Tenesmus
Trigeminal	– Facial

Epidural morphine should usually be considered before more invasive or destructive nerve blocking procedures. It can be effective for leg, arm or trunk pain. The level of the epidural injection is not critical because the morphine diffuses into the CSF and circulates to cover all the spinal opioid receptors (*see Spinal Drugs*).

Clinical principles of using nerve blocks include:

- Explain carefully
- Stop warfarin
- Use local anaesthetic before neurolytics
- The procedure should be painless
- Monitor morphine dose afterwards

Explanation is essential. Nerve blocks are usually performed by an anaesthetist specializing in pain clinic work. Discuss with the patient and family, explaining potential benefits and also any risks. If the patient is dubious it is best postponed. It can be a difficult decision for a patient who has adjusted psychologically to having no further interventions. Warfarin must be stopped or reversed before the procedure (*see Bleeding*). Anti-coagulants are a contra-indication to a nerve block, because of the risk of haemorrhage. Local anaesthetic should be given first, to cause a reversible block, to see the effect on the pain, and any side-effects, before a permanent neurolytic block is given. Sometimes pain relief following a local anaesthetic block can last weeks or months (for unknown reasons). Bupivacaine (Marcain) is usually used. The maximum safe dose is 1ml of 0.25%\kg\4 hours, i.e. well above the usual dose of 20ml 8-12 hourly for most procedures. (10ml of 0.25% Marcain is 25mg). The procedure itself should be painless. This is particularly important in this group of patients, who have often already suffered a great deal of physical discomfort, and who are being promised the hope of increased comfort. Use plenty of local anaesthetic, and wait for it to work. IV midazolam can be used for sedation, which causes retrograde amnesia. Stop morphine after the procedure, and observe for 24 hours. This is to avoid respiratory depression. Morphine requirements fall if the pain is reduced by the nerve block, and the previous correct dose of morphine is then too high, and may cause severe drowsiness or even respiratory depression. If pain starts to recur, re-start morphine at 5mg 4 hourly, and increase the dose as necessary (*see Morphine*). A less severe pain may be unmasked by the successful nerve block of the most painful area.

Coeliac Plexus Block (CPB) is a very sucessful technique, particularly in cancers of:

- Pancreas
- Stomach
- Liver

CPB will often control epigastric or back pains that have not been controlled by morphine. At least 80% of patients get good pain relief, and in only 5% does the technique fail to reduce pain levels. The effect usually lasts 12 months, and it can therefore be considered permanent in the terminally ill. The procedure is performed bilaterally under intravenous sedation and local anaesthetic, and under X-ray control, in order to position the needle. A 15cm needle is inserted 7cm from the mid-line, below the 12th rib. The plexus lies behind the peritoneum, at the level of L1, just anterior to the aorta (which is just anterior to the body of the L1 vertebra). 50ml of 50% alcohol are injected as a neurolytic (enough to cause intoxication for a few hours afterwards). Absence of post-block hypotension indicates failure of the technique. Side-effects include postural hypotension for 1-2 days, backache for a few hours, increased gut motility (diarrhoea) and a hangover for a few hours (if absolute alcohol is used). Rare complications include retroperitoneal haematoma (from aorta or IVC), L1 neuritis (numbness on the anterior thigh), pneumothorax, paraplegia (injection into spinal artery) and kidney puncture. CPB can also be performed at open laparotomy, providing the plexus is not obscured by tumour, or via an anterior approach under CT scan control.

Reference: Hanna M *et al.* (1989) The use of coeliac plexus blockade in patients with chronic pain, Palliative Medicine; 4: 11-16.

Paravertebral thoracic block can be useful for:

- chest wall pain
- mesothelioma
- vertebral metastases
- rib fractures
- post-thoracotomy pain

A paravertebral block has the advantage over intercostal blocks that it covers several dermatomal segments. 15ml of 0.25% bupivacaine normally covers at least 4 segments. After a diagnostic block with bupivacaine, a longer-lasting block can be achieved by inserting 5ml of aqueous phenol. It can safely be repeated if pain control is not satisfactory. Complications are rare. Although called a somatic block, it probably involves the sympathetic fibres which run nearby, and it can be used for oesophageal pain (T3,4,5). Proceedure: The needle is inserted (with or without X-ray control) into the paravertebral space which lies anterior to the transverse processes, and communicates with the epidural space via the intervertebral foramina.

Reference: Eason MJ, Wyatt R (1979) Paravertebral thoracic block -a re-appraisal. Anaesthesia; 34: 638-642).

Intercostal blocks are useful for rib pain, from a metastasis or fracture. Under local anaesthetic an injection of 1ml 5% phenol can be given at the posterior angle of the rib, (the neurovascular bundle runs inferior to each rib). If performed too anteriorly, the lateral cutaneous branch can be missed. Multiple intercostal blocks (using either phenol or cryotherapy or radio-frequency coagulation) can be used instead of paravertebral block for chest wall pain.

Local steroid injection can be useful for rib or vertebral pain. Intralesional methylprednisolone (Depomedrone) 40mg injected into the rib periosteum, under intercostal block, is a simple technique which relieves pain due to a rib metastasis in 70% within 2-10 days and is an alternative to radiotherapy for patients not well enough to attend the radiotherapy department. Epidural methlyprednisolone plus bupivacaine can reduce to pain of a vertebral metastasis.

Reference: Rowell NP (1988) Intralesional methylprednisolone for rib metastasis: an alternative to radiotherapy? Palliative Medicine; 2: 153-155.

Brachial plexus infusion is occasionally indicated for severe nerve pain in the arm, usually due to a Pancoast tumour or nodes in the axilla. A catheter is inserted (via the supraclavicular, interscalene or axillary route) and left in place. 20ml of 0.5% bupivacaine should produce analgesia within 10 minutes. A 20ml injection is given because this is about the volume of the sheath that covers the brachial plexus. If the concentration of the local anaesthetic is reduced, by diluting with normal saline (0.25%, 0.125%, 0.0625%) the motor blockade can be reduced, so that movement may return to the arm, without the pain returning. The local anaesthetic can be given as bolus injections, 20ml every 8 hours (when a relative may need to be taught how to give the injections if the patient goes home) or by continuous infusion by pump using a Graseby MS26A. For unknown reasons the effect of local anaesthetic can sometimes be long-lasting, so it is worthwhile stopping the infusions from time to time (leaving the catheter in place) to see if the pain has stopped. Neurolytic blocks are contra-indicated in the arm, because some patients find the numb heavy arm more unpleasant than the pain, and also because there is a high incidence of painful neuritis at this site following neurolytic blocks.

Reference: Clark AJ, Simpson KH, Ellis FR (1990) Continuous brachial plexus block in the management of intractable cancer pain in the arm, Palliative Medicine; 4: 123-125.

Hip Block is useful for painful metastases or fractures in the head of femur or acetabulum, where a patient is not fit enough for radiotherapy or internal fixation. A block with bupivacaine can sometimes reduce pain for several weeks. The technique is described in the reference.

Reference: James CDT, Little TF (1976) Regional hip blockade – a simplified technique for the relief of intractable osteoarthritic pain, Anaesthesia; 31: 1060-1067)

Intrathecal phenol may be useful for the control of somatic perineal pain, from local spread of cancer (but not for referred visceral or nerve pain) that is not controlled by morphine. However, there is a significant risk of leg weakness, urinary and faecal incontinence following the procedure, and it is best reserved for patients who already have a colostomy and indwelling catheter, and who have already tried epidural morphine, and where the risk of leg weakness is understood. In one study of 9 patients only moderate pain pain relief was obtained for a short duration (less than 3 weeks), but other studies show that excellent pain relief for several months can occasionally be obtained in individual patients. The injection is given slowly via the L5\S1 interspace, using heavy bupivacaine initially for a trial and if the pain is controlled it is repeated using 0.3-1ml of phenol in glycerine. The spread of the neurolytic is controlled by gravity. The patient is positioned sitting and leaning back at 45 degrees during the procedure, so that the anterior (motor) nerve roots are rotated away from the neurolytic, to minimize the risk of motor paralysis.

Reference:
Lynch J, Zech D, Grand S. The role of intrathecal neurolysis in the treatment of cancer-related peri-anal and perineal pain. Palliative Medicine 1992; 6: 140-145.

Lumbar sympathetic block can help to relieve tenesmus. It should be performed bilaterally. It should also be considered for control of pain in the legs if there is a burning pain or a hyperaesthetic element to the pain, suggesting damage to sympathetic pain fibres, when the leg is usually also cold with trophic skin changes (shiny taut skin, hair loss, areas of hyperkeratosis).

Trigeminal block can be useful for facial pain that is not being controlled by morphine. The Gasserian ganglion can be blocked using a radiofrequency thermocoagulation technique or individual branches can be blocked with small amounts of absolute alcohol. There is no motor blockade and the effect is long-lasting. NB A throbbing facial pain that is not controlled by morphine may be due to an abscess, when the WBC count may not raised, and the pain often settles with a broad-spectrum antibiotic.

Specialized techniques that are rarely indicated, include:

- Cordotomy
- Pituitary ablation

Cordotomy (tractotomy) means destruction of pain fibres in the spinal cord. It is only indicated for severe unilateral pain, below C5, unresponsive to other treatments, in a patient with advanced cancer. 80% get pain relief, but at the cost of unilateral numbness and sometimes a weak leg. The effect lasts about 6 months. The patient has to be able to co-operate during the procedure. It is performed percutaneously with a needle inserted at C1-C2, (below the mastoid process) under Xray control. When the needle is in place an electric current is used to produce a heat lesion.

Pituitary ablation (hypophysectomy) was recognized in 1953 to reduce pain from bone metastases. It is a relatively simple technique performed under general anaesthetic. It is less effective than cordotomy; only 40% get complete pain relief and the effect can wear off after a few weeks. There is a high morbidity, with a risk of visual field defects and CSF rhinorrhoea. Hormone replacement therapy is needed afterwards (cortisone, and sometimes thyroxine and desmopressin). It has been virtually replaced by the LHRH analogues which in effect cause a chemical hypophysectomy.

Some Anatomy:

Peripheral nerves are mixed motor and sensory nerves, and comprise the cranial nerves and 30 pairs of spinal nerves:

SPINAL NERVES		
8 Cervical	–	head and arm
12 Thoracic	–	chest abdomen
5 Lumbar	–	front of leg
5 Sacral	–	back of leg, perineum, scrotum

Peripheral nerve blocks can cause weakness, as well as pain relief. Chest wall weakness is not so important, so intercostal blocks are useful to relieve chest wall pain. Peripheral nerves can be blocked by:

- Radio-frequency coagulation (heat lesion)
- Chemical neurolytics (alcohol, phenol)
- Cryoprobe (cold lesion)

Radio-frequency is the preferred method of blocking because the effect is more reliable than cryoprobe, it lasts several months, and it is less likely to cause painful neuritis, which can develop after neurolytics. A stimulating current is used to locate the nerve and then a high frequency current is used to coagulate it.

Visceral pain fibres from the internal organs travel with the sympathetic fibres, and therefore blocks of the sympathetic fibres or plexuses (stellate, coeliac or lumbar) can also control pain. Pain fibres from the visceral organs run with the sympathetic fibres as follows:

VISCERAL PAIN FIBRES	
T2-5	Lungs
T4-5	Oesophagus
T6-8	Stomach, Pancreas, Liver
T9-10	Small bowel
T10	Ovaries, Testes
T10-L3	Colon
T11-L1	Bladder
S2-S5	Prostate

The posterior nerve roots that enter the spinal cord, consist of sensory fibres that have separated from the motor fibres of the mixed peripheral nerve, before they enter the spinal cord. They can be selectively destroyed by a dorsal rhizotomy. Another way of selectively destroying these sensory pain fibres in the posterior root is by using intrathecal phenol to destroy them as they pass through the CSF, before they enter the spinal cord. Epidural local anaesthetic diffuses onto both the sensory and motor nerve roots and therefore also causes motor weakness, as well as pain relief.

In the posterior horn of the spinal cord the pain fibres synapse with spinal nerve fibres. Endogenous opioids act here (in the descending inhibitory pathways from the midbrain). Morphine acts at this point, so spinal morphine does not cause any motor weakness or postural hypotension, unlike local anaesthetics (see Spinal drugs).

The antero-lateral tracts carry pain fibres that have crossed over in the cord from the other side of the body before they pass up to the thalamus. They can be interrupted by a cordotomy which causes numbness to the opposite side of the body.

Further Reading:
Wells JCD (1989) The use of nerve destruction for relief of pain in cancer: a review. Palliative Medicine; 3: 239-247.
Hardy PAJ (1990) The role of the pain clinic in the management of the terminally ill. British Journal of Hospital Medicine; 43: 142-146.

NERVE PAIN

Nerve pain can be defined as burning or stabbing pain in an area of altered sensation. It is difficult to treat and responds only partially to morphine. It is has the following characteristics:

- Burning or stabbing
- Variable (with time of day, position, mood)
- Light touch may be painful (despite numbness)
- Disturbs sleep
- Worsened by emotonal upset

The common clinical causes of nerve pain are brachial plexus damage (C8, T1) causing arm pain usually due to an apical lung cancer (Pancoast's syndrome) or malignant nodes in the axilla or supraclavicular fossa from breast cancer, or lumbo-sacral plexus damage causing leg pain usually due to recurrent pelvic tumour (*see Pelvic Recurrence*).

The mechanism of nerve pain is not understood, hence the befuddled terminology with many different words (neuropathic pain, neuropathy, neuritis, neuralgia, causalgia and de-afferentation pain) all used to describe the syndrome of burning or stabbing pain with hyperaesthesia (increased sensitivity) or dysaesthesia (unpleasant tingling). The pain is not transmitted via the activation of nerve endings (hence the term de-afferentation pain) but due to damage of peripheral nerves which causes spontaneous electical activity and also, after 1-2 months, permanent changes in the activity of neurones in the dorsal horn of the cord which perpetuates the pain ("pain memory"). Damage at higher levels in the cord or brain can produce a similar pattern of pain ("central pain"). The pain does not appear to be transmitted via opioid-sensitive synapses. Drug treatments aim to alter the abnormal neural activity by influencing neuro-transmission. Since there are several different mechanisms involved, the responses to treatment are, not suprisingly, variable. Further research is needed.

Management steps in nerve pain:

- Explanation
- Morphine
- Steroids
- Tricyclic
- Anticonvulsant
- Other drugs
- TENS
- Nerve blocks
- Elevate pain threshold (emotional element)

Explanation helps the patient, who may fear that such a severe pain automatically means that the cancer is spreading. The pain is due to nerve irritation (not spread of cancer) and it does not respond to ordinary pain-killers. A step-by step approach and the first step is a good night's sleep. It is always possible to reduce the pain, if not abolish it.

Morphine is the first step, and often helps to reduce the pain, especially the aching element, and <u>may</u> partially control the stabbing or burning pain. The dose must be carefully balanced so that the pain is reduced as much as possible without causing too much drowsiness. In one study 28 patients with nerve pain were given an IV infusion of opioid and 21 experienced more than 50% pain relief, although some of the effect may have been due to sedation (Portnoy *et al.* 1990).

Steroids should be considered (dexamethasone 8mg a day) especially for nerve pain of recent onset, when nerve compression may still be partially reversible. Further rationale for using steroids is that the early treatment of nerve pain may prevent the central changes in the spinal cord, which seem to perpetuate and worsen the pain. For example, analgesia given prior to amputation can reduce the development of phantom limb pain later.

Tricyclics are important, especially if there is a <u>burning</u> element to the pain, and seem to have a centrally-acting analgesic effect for certain types of nerve pain, (but have not been shown to have any analgesic effect for non-neuropathic pain). The analgesic effect seems to be distinct from any anti-depressant effect. The analgesic effect occurs more quickly, in 2-3 days, and at lower doses and plasma levels than the anti-depressant effect. <u>Tricyclics</u> are thought to increase the activity of the descending inhibitory fibres by increasing spinal levels of noradrenaline (by blocking its re-uptake at the synapse). Amitriptyline 25-100mg a day, has been shown to control nerve pain in about 40% of cases. In one controlled study (McQuay 1993) 75mg amitriptyline produced significantly greater pain control than 25 or 50mg (but also a greater incidence of dry mouth and drowsiness). Newer anti-depressants (lofepramine, dothiepin) may be as effective as amitriptyline or imipramine, and may have fewer side-effects .

<u>Crossover studies</u> have demonstrated the analgesic effect of tricyclics, but have been mainly done on non-malignant pain and only involve small numbers of patients. 16 out of 24 patients with post-herpetic neuralgia had a

good or excellent response to amitriptyline, in a median dose of 75mg, which was significantly better than placebo and effective for both burning and stabbing pains (Watson *et al* 1982). In 2 double-blind studies in painful diabetic neuropathy, 8 out of 12 patients had pain relief with amitriptyline or imipramine 100mg at night (Turkington 1980) and in another study 7 out of 12 patients improved on imipramine 100mg at night with no improvements on placebo (Kvinesdal *et al* 1984).

Anti-convulsants are membrane-stabilizing drugs that reduce neuronal activity in various ways, and are particularly indicated if there is a stabbing element to the pain. They have been used since the recognition that 80% of patients with trigeminal neuralgia respond to phenytoin or carbamazapine within a few days. Sodium valproate (Epilim), 200-600mg TID, is the drug of first choice. It significantly reduces the pain in about 20% of patients. Carmbimazole (Tegretol) 100-400mg BD, is an alternative, but can cause drowsiness or dizziness, and should be started in a low dose and increased gradually every 1-2 days. Phenytoin 300mg nocte or and Clonazepam 0.5-2mg daily are also effective, but clonazepam can cause excessive drowsiness. A comparative study of 170 patients with shooting pains from a variety of causes showed clonazepam helped 41% and phenytoin, carbamazepine and valproate 15% (Swerdlow and Cundill 1981).

Crossover studies have shown carbamezepine 600mg daily was effective in 28 out of 30 patients with diabetic neuropathy (Rull *et al* 1969). In other studies phenytoin was significantly more effective than placebo for painful neuropathy in diabetes and Fabry's disease (Chadda and Mathur 1978, Lockman *et al.* 1973).

Other drugs that may have a place, and have been found to have some analgesic properties for various sorts of pains include flecainide, clonidine, baclofen, IV naloxone and IV physostigmine. Flecainide (Tambocor), 100-200mg BD, can be tried if the above drugs fail to control pain. It is a membrane-stabilizing drug normally used in cardiac arrythmias, that has been shown to help some cases of malignant nerve pain. It should not be used with a history of cardiac arrythmias nor with tricyclics, which may increase the liklihood of arrythmias. Clonidine is an agonist at the a-adrenergic receptors of the sympathetic system and has been reported to reduce pain in diabetic neuropathy and to increase sensitivity to opioids in neuropathic pain, and may be of value when given spinally, by mimicking noradrenaline and inhibiting pain transmission.

TENS can occasionally help, but the effect is short-lived and in some patients can aggrevate the pain. Multi-channel machines may prove more helpful (*see TENS*).

Nerve blocks with local anaesthetic can sometimes be useful for initial assessment of the pain, to see if there is an element of peripheral nerve damage. Neurolytic blocks are a last resort, and are generally avoided, since the pain is due to nerve damage, and further nerve damage may aggrevate the pain. A brachial plexus infusion of bupivacaine or an epidural infusion of bupivacaine and\or morphine may be necessary for severe uncontrolled pains (*see Nerve blocks, Spinal drugs*). If there is burning pain with evidence of sympathetic damage (purplish discolouration, smooth hairless skin, increased sweating, skin tenderness) then a sympathetic nerve block is indicated, using a stellate ganglion block for pain in the arm or a bilateral lumbar sympathetic block for the leg.

Raising the pain threshold. The emotional element of pain, so often over-looked, can be the secret to the successful management of nerve pain, which is often worsened by emotional distress. Management should involve:

- Good quality sleep
- Emotional counselling
- Practical support
- Social diversions
- Relaxation therapy
- Spiritual support

Referal to a psychologist may help if the patient understands and accepts that emotional counselling can help control pain (*see Psychological support*).

References:
McQuay HJ, Pharmacological treatment of neuralgic and neuropathic pain. Cancer Surveys Vol 7, No 1, 1988.
Portnoy RK, Foley KM, Inturrisi CE, The nature of opioid responsiveness and its implications for neuropathic pain: new hypotheses derived from studies of opioid infusions. Pain 1990; 43: 273-286.
McQuay HJ, Carroll D, Glynn CJ. Dose-response for analgesic effect of amitriptyline in chronic pain. Anaesthesia 1993; 48: 281–285.

NSAIDs

Non-steroidal anti-inflammatory drugs (NSAIDs) block prostaglandin synthesis by inhibiting the enzyme cyclo-oxygenase. NSIADs are mainly used to control bone pain, but other uses are in sweating and bladder spasms.

Naproxen (Naprosyn) 500mg BD is a useful first-choice NSAID. It is available as tablets, suspension or suppositories. It is a phenylproprionate. Alternative NSAIDs are needed, because:

- Only 60% respond to any NSAID
- 20% respond on changing the NSAID
- 20% do not respond

Alternatives NSAIDs of different chemical groups are:

- diclofenac (Voltarol) – acetic acid
- piroxicam (Feldene) – oxicam
- ketoprofen (Oruvail) – proprionic acid
- diflunisal (Dolobid) – aspirin derivative
- indomethacin (Indocid) – indole derivative

Diclofenac, 50mg BD, is available as a dispersible tablet. Piroxicam 10-40mg has the advantage of a long half-life (40-80 hours) and is given as a single daily dose. Ketoprofen is also available as a single daily dose, Oruvail 200mg, being a slow-release preparation of a short half-life drug (2-4 hours) and it is therefore safer than piroxicam in the elderly. Diflunisal, 500mg BD, is a non-acetylated salicylate and is useful if the platelet count is low, as it does not affect platelet function or bleeding time. Indomethacin, 50mg QID (100mg suppository BD) is the most potent of the NSAIDs, although the slow-release capsule, 75mg BD, is about the same potency as naproxen.

Weak NSAIDs include: ibuprofen (Brufen, Fenbid), mefanamic acid (Ponstan) and tolmetin (Tolectin).

Side-effects of NSAIDs are a reason to change to a different NSAID, because they may not occur with an NSAID of a different group. They include:

- Dyspepsia – 20%
- Fluid retention
- Gastric ulceration
- Asthma may be worsened
- Headaches (indomethacin)
- Diarrhoea (mefenamic acid)
- Reduced platelet function (rare)
- Renal function may be worsened (rare)

Gastric irritation can be reduced by ranitidine misoprostol or omeprazole (*see Heartburn*). Misoprostol 200 micrograms BD to QID prevents mucosal injury by NSAIDs and may be used if there is a previous history of peptic ulceration. It seems to protect against both gastric and duodenal ulceration. Healing of established ulcers while on NSIADs is probably best achieved by high dose ranitidine. The drugs that protect against ulceration do not always stop the dyspepsia.

Topical NSAIDs are rubbed in as gels, and some patients find them helpful, even though they produce only one fifth the plasma level of an oral dose of the same drug. They include:

- diclofenac (Voltarol) gel
- piroxicam (Feldene) gel
- felbinac (Traxam) gel

Subcutaneous NSAIDs. Diclofenac (Voltarol) 150–300mg per 24 hours (75mg per 3ml ampoule) and ketorolac (Toradol) 60–90mg per 24 hours (10mg per 1ml ampoule) can both be given by SC infusion. Both need a separate syringe driver. Ketorolac is a new NSAID which may have a place in the treatment of opioid non-responsive pain.

OEDEMA

Oedema means excessive accumulation of tissue fluid. Ankle swelling is the commonest problem. Oedema is usually due to a combination of factors:

- Low serum albumin
- Drugs causing fluid retention (NSAIDs, steroids)
- Reduced mobility
- Heart failure
- Venous thrombosis (*see DVT*)
- Lymphatic obstruction (*see Lymphoedema*)

Treatment options for oedema include:

- Diuretics
- Stop drugs
- Exercise
- Elevate legs
- Support stockings

Diuretics cause a diuresis which may be more troublesome than the ankle swelling. Walking and muscular contractions increases the venous circulation, and immobility is a major cause of ankle swelling. Leg elevation is effective for 1-2 hours, but more effective if combined with a mild diuretic. Diuretics reduce sodium reabsorbtion by the renal tubules and increase urine output. Useful diuretics include:

Bendrofluazide 5-10mg daily is a thiazide and a mild diuretic.

Frusemide 40-80mg daily is a loop diuretic that causes a diuresis within 1 hour that lasts 6 hours. Much higher doses are needed if there is renal failure. It should be given early in the day so the diuresis does not disturb sleep (unimportant if the patient is catheterized). The problems include excessive diuresis, hypokalaemia or hypotension.

Metolozone 5-20mg daily is a thiazide, which is a potent diuretic when combined with frusemide. It is useful for oedema that is resistant to frusemide alone.

Amiloride 5-10mg daily is a mild potassium-sparing diuretic that can be added to a longterm regime of frusemide to prevent hypokalaemia, and is easier to take than potassium supplements.

Spironolactone is an aldosterone antagonist that is useful for the treatment of ascites (*see Ascites*).

OESOPHAGEAL CANCER

Oesophageal cancer causes about 5600 deaths per year in the UK. It typically presents with dysphagia and weight loss. Intermittent heartburn can occur, but constant pain suggests that the tumour is already far-advanced. It is more common in smokers. The prognosis is very poor. The tumour is usually advanced at presentation, and few patients survive more than 6 months from diagnosis.

Diagnosis is by barium swallow, endoscopy and biopsy, and CT scan to assess nodal involvement. Surgery and radical radiotherapy both have poor results (only 5% survive 5 years).

Surgery has a 10% mortality, and is only attempted in relatively fit patients with no evidence of metastases. With lower third resections, the stomach can be mobilized and pulled up to anastomose with the oesophagus (gastric pull-through), with middle third resections a segment of colon is used to form a pseudo-oesophagus (colonic transposition). Both operations restore swallowing, but 30% of patients come to need dilations of the anastomosis. Upper third tumours can only be treated by radiotherapy. Radical radiotherapy (50-60 Gy over 6 weeks) can be given for squamous tumours (90%) but adenocarcinomas (10%) are relatively radio-resistant.

Palliative radiotherapy (3000cGy over 2 weeks) and\or palliative bypass surgery (gastro-oesophageal anastomosis or using a segment of colon to bypass the tumour) can sometimes relieve or prevent malignant strictures and improve swallowing in advanced disease.

Metastases occur to nodes in the mediastinum (and neck), and later to liver, lung, bone, brain and skin. There is no effective chemotherapy for this tumour, which is restricted to clinical trials.

Problems in advanced cancer of the oesophagus include:

- Pain
- Dysphagia
- Hoarseness
- Tube problems
- Fistula into the trachea

Pain may be due to heartburn in the early stages, but continuous pain (retrosternal, or between the shoulder blades) is due to visceral cancer pain, and requires morphine. A change in the pattern of pain, with intermittent exacerbations, may be due to infiltration of a vertebra or the pleura.

Dysphagia can be due to a benign stricture, due to a surgical anastomosis or post-radiation, and most patients who have had surgery or RT need dilatations ("stretches") every few months afterwards. Early strictures can be improved by simple dilatation, but a tube should be inserted whenever possible. Laser therapy can improve swallowing even in advanced disease.

Tube problems include blockage, or displacement or disintegration (*see Dysphagia*).

Hoarseness is due to recurrent laryngeal nerve damage (*see Hoarseness*).

Arrythmias can occur due to pericardial involvement, and can usually be controlled with digoxin or beta-blockers.

Tracheo-oesophageal fistula formation causes coughing after drinking. It can be confirmed by a coloured drink, which stains the sputum. It is a terminal event, and the patient is unlikely to live for more than a few days. A small fistula in a relatively fit patient can sometimes be managed by inserting a Nottingham tube or possibly a prosthesis (Cancer 1988; 61: 1679-84).

ORGAN DONATION

Organ donation can sometimes be a comforting idea to both the patient and the relatives. Malignancy is generally thought of as a contra-indication to organ donation except for corneas, but heart valves can also be donated, and patients with proven primary brain tumours can donate kidneys.

Written consent should be obtained from the patient whenever possible, but verbal consent from the next of-kin is the only legal requirement in the UK (ideally witnessed by 2 members of staff). Permission from the coroner is needed if the death would normally have been reported.

Screening should be performed before death for Hepatitis B and HIV.

Corneas can be donated by cancer patients of any age, provided there is no history of eye damage or surgery. Motor neurone disease is also a contra-indication (because the cause remains unknown). The eyes need to be taken within 24 hours of death. Contact the local opthalmology department. After enucleation the eye sockets can be packed and the eyelids stitched down to look normal.

Kidneys can be donated by patients under 70 with histologically proven primary brain tumours. The Regional Transplant Co-ordinator must be involved. The kidneys need to be removed within an hour of death. The family can be present after death for a few minutes. The removed kidneys are perfused with ice-cold preserving fluid and then stored in ice. The spleen is also removed for tissue typing. The family can see the body after death (there is only a transverse abdominal scar). Contra-indications include chronic renal disease or septicaemia. Previous medical illnesses or a reduced fluid intake or urine output prior to death need not preclude the use of kidneys for transplantation. The patient does not need to be on a life-support machine before death. Most kidneys for transplant are from ventilated patients with brain stem death, but kidney donation following asystole is possible. In a series of 12 patients with primary brain tumours who became asystolic kidney donors there were 24 transplants and 12 longterm functioning grafts (Peters and Sutcliffe, 1992).

Heart valves (aortic and pulmonary) can be donated and used for transplantation if the patient is under 60, providing there is no malignant invasion of the heart. They should be taken within 72 hours of death and can be stored for up to 5 years before transplant.

Reference:
Peters D, Sutcliffe J. Organ donation: the hospice perspective. Palliative Medicine 1992; 6: 212-216.

OVARIAN CANCER

Ovarian cancer causes around 4,000 deaths per year in the UK, and accounts for 6% of cancer deaths in women. It presents typically with abdominal distension. The tumour is usually far advanced at presentation and prognosis is often poor. Most are adenocarcinomas. 5% of cases are familial, possibly dominantly inherited, and screening with transvaginal ultrasound should be considered for such families.

Treatment aims to surgically debulk as much tumour as possible. Only 20% of patients present with stage 1 disease, treated with TAH and BSO, when 67% survive 5 years. Radiotherapy or chemotherapy are used if spread has occured to pelvic or para-aortic nodes or into the peritoneum as seedlings, when survival can be prolonged for 1-2 years but very few patients are cured. The place of abdominal RT is not clear, and it is used less frequently now.

Chemotherapy with carboplatin is as effective as combinations of drugs. A large international trial is currently comparing carboplatin with the much more toxic combination of Cisplatin, doxorubicin and cyclophosphamide. The initial aim may still be cure if peritoneal seedlings are small. Treatment is monitored by CT scan and ultrasound scan. Plasma CA 125 levels provide additional information if raised. It is usually continued for 6 cycles if the patient responds. If there is no response after 3 cycles of treatment it should be stopped. There is no useful second line chemotherapy. Elderly patients are not suitable for vigourous chemotherapy but chlorambucil 5mg daily for 14 days a month can give useful palliation in patients who have been too ill or frail for the platinum analogues, and about 30% get some response, with reduced abdominal masses or ascites.

Metastases are unusual but can occur to liver, lung, CNS or marrow.

Intra-peritoneal radio-labelled monoclonal antibody therapy may come to have a place in treatment. In one study 4 out of 16 patients with minimal peritoneal disease had remissions for 8 months to 3 years. Newer techniques with high radiation yttrium–90 instead of I–131 may produce better results.

Problems in advanced cancer of the ovary include:

- Ascites
- Pleural effusions
- Intestinal obstruction (25%)

Reference: Williams C, Current issues in cancer, Br Med J 1992; 304: 1501-4.

PAIN

Pain is defined as an unpleasant sensory and emotional experience. A useful clinical definition is that pain is what the patient says hurts.

Pain control can occur at several levels:

- Nerve ending   NSAID
- Peripheral nerve   Nerve block
- Dorsal horn   Opioids
- Spino thalamic tract   Cordotomy
- Midbrain   Opioids
- Cortex   General anaesthetic

Cancer pain is experienced by 70% of cancer patients, but 30% do not get pain related to their cancer. It is more common in some cancers, such as pancreas and oesophagus (80-90%) than others such as lymphoma (less than 50%). 90% of cancer pains can be controlled with simple methods, and expertise has reached a point where all cancer patients can expect to be free of pain. 1% of cancer pain, however, remains difficult to control. Cancer pain can be classified into:

- Visceral
- Soft tissue
- Bone
- Nerve
- Secondary visceral spasm (gut, bladder, rectum)

Assessment of cancer pain is often straightforward, and based on the patient's verbal report of the pain (see table). The description of the pain usually gives a clear indication of the type of cancer pain: Continuous pain (visceral or soft tissue) usually responds well to morphine. Pain on movement (bone pain) responds poorly to morphine, but is usually controlled by radiotherapy or NSAIDs. Stabbing or burning pain (nerve pain) responds partially to morphine, and usually needs tricyclics or anti-convulsants as well. Colicky pain that comes and goes may be due to treatable constipation or may respond to anti-spasmodics.

A body chart, drawn with, or by, the patient is a useful communication tool when assessing pain, which allows the patient to communicate in detail and makes the pain "visible", demonstrating the sites of pains (80% have two or more pains) and makes a record for the notes. Body charts are useful for initial assessment, but should not be used for intractable pain, because it can focus on rather than distract from the pain.

CANCER PAINS		
DESCRIPTION OF PAIN	CLASSIFICATION OF PAIN	TREATMENT OF PAIN
"Continuous"	Visceral or Soft tissue	Morphine
"On movement"	Bone	RT or NSAIDs
"Stabbing or Burning"	Nerve	Morphine Tricyclics Anti-convulsants Steroids
"Comes and goes"	Colic	Anti-spasmodic

Detailed assessment of each pain includes:
- Site
- Severity
- Timing (When does it occur?)
- Quality (What is it like?)
- Radiation (Does it move anywhere?)
- Provoking factors (what makes it worse?)
- Relieving factors (What improves it?)
  - Position
  - Mood
  - Analgesics
  - Radiotherapy
  - Nerve blocks

Analgesic history is essential (and often forgotten): The analgesics actually being swallowed are very often different to those prescribed – discuss in detail and inspect the medicine bottles. If the pain has responded even partially to an opioid drug, then it is usually possible to get complete pain relief with a carefully titrated dose of morphine. Ask about:

- Analgesics tried
- Doses
- When taken
- For how long
- How effective
- Side-effects

Monitoring pain control is the key to good management. The aim is a pain-free patient. Ask daily about pain severity. The best assessment of pain severity is the patient's verbal report. <u>Pain scores</u> are a direct and simple way to monitor pain control. The patient is asked 3 times a day to rate the severity of pain on a score of 0-10, where 0 is no pain at all and 10 is the worst pain imaginable. The scores are recorded on a chart. <u>Indirect assessment</u> of pain control can be made from:

- Activity
- Mobility
- Sleep
- Analgesic requirements

Non-malignant pains (due to incidental medical conditions) account for around 15% of pains in cancer patients and will not respond to morphine. Without a careful history they can be mistaken for cancer pains. They include:

- Tension headache
- Arthritis
- Frozen shoulder
- Angina
- Oesophagitis
- Peptic ulcer
- Anal fissure
- Renal colic
- Scar pain
- Vincristine neuropathy

Morphine-responsiveness is the key question in managing cancer pain. Some pains are completely responsive, typically visceral and soft tissue pains, others are only partially responsive such as nerve pains, and some are not responsive such as the incident pain on movement due to bone metastases. Some pains can be called morphine-irrelevant, when the patient complains bitterly of physical pain as a way of communicating their mental anguish (*see Spiritual pain*).

Visceral\soft tissue pain is continuous aching pain than typically responds well to morphine. Nerve endings occur in the capsule of the liver or kidney, and in the muscles of the small intestines. Pain is due to distension or traction on visceral organs, such as by adhesions. Mild visceral pains may respond to paracetamol or co-proxamol, which should be tried first, but morphine is usually needed as pain increases, and the morphine dose must be titrated (i.e. start low and increase until painfree). Visceral pain can be severe, even overwhelming and yet the patient may appear quiet and withdrawn and depressed, completely unlike the typical picture of acute pain.

Visceral pain that does not respond to morphine is unusual and is an indication to review the patient's pains, and to reassess the morphine dose and consider a nerve block. <u>Morphine dose may be too low</u>. 10% of patients on morphine need high doses, and 1% need very high doses. If the morphine has helped a bit and the patient is not drowsy the rule is to increase the dose. Poor morphine absorbtion may be the problem if the patient has had recent abdominal surgery, or has severe diarrhoea. Change to a subcutaneous infusion of diamorphine. It is possible that in some patients morphine does not diffuse properly into the CSF, in which case spinal morphine would be effective when oral or subcutaneous morphine are not (see *Spinal drugs*). Anxiety is a common factor in pain, and a persistent visceral pain that is not responding to well-titrated doses of morphine may respond by adding chlorpromazine 12.5-25mg 8 hourly or haloperidol 1.5-5mg 12 hourly. Nerve blocks may be required if continuous pain does not respond to morphine. In this case, increasing the dose of morphine makes the patient drowsy, without controlling the pain. The commonest visceral pains that do not respond completely to morphine, and require a nerve block are pancreatic (coeliac plexus block) and chest wall pain (intercostal or paravertebral block). (*see Nerve blocks*). Radiotherapy or chemotherapy may occasionally help in pain control by reducing tumour bulk. Chest pain from a large bronchial tumour may be controlled. Renal pain can be controlled by radiotherapy if the contra- lateral kidney is functioning. Early compression of a nerve plexus may be reversed. Infection in soft tissue (especially in head and neck cancers) can cause a severe pain that will not respond to morphine (see below).

Infection can cause severe continuous pain, that will not respond to morphine, but will respond to antibiotics. This is described especially in tumours of the head and neck. In one study, (Bruera, 1986) 7 patients with head and neck tumours had severe chronic pain that responded quickly to antibiotics. Such tumours are often ulcerated and necrotic and surrounded by swelling and erythema. However fever is often absent and the WBC count is not always elevated if the patient is already on steroids. The pain is sometimes described as having a throbbing element. The pain does not respond to morphine but will respond to an antibiotic. Infection should always be suspected in patients with advanced cancer of the head and neck who have a changing pattern of pain, and a therapeutic trial of a broad-spectrum antibiotic such as chloramphenicol or Co-amoxiclav (Augmentin) should be tried.

Liver pain is a common visceral pain that deserves special description. Nevertheless, it only occurs in about 40% of patients with liver metastases. It is due to stretching of the liver capsule (the liver parenchyma has no pain fibres). It causes a deep aching pain in the right upper quadrant of the abdomen, right side and back, often worsened by prolonged walking or standing up. Occasionally the pain is left-sided or epigastric. Gastric compression can cause discomfort after meals. It is usually well controlled by morphine. Slow enlargement of the liver can be painless. Liver pain that does not respond to morphine is almost always controlled by a coeliac plexus block (*see nerve blocks*). Liver embolization (injection of an artery with a chemical to cause infarct of part of the liver) is sometimes used for control of liver cancer, but should rarely be used for pain control, as it is a very painful preceedure in itself, and not always effective (*see Interventional radiology*).

Sub-capsular haemorrhage can cause a sudden increase in pain due to sudden stretching of the liver capsule, and this requires an increase in morphine dose for 2-3 days (sometimes a large increase) which can be reduced again as the pain settles (when the patient will begin to become drowsy).

Bone pain is worse on movement, relieved by rest, with bony tenderness. The treatment of choice is palliative radiotherapy. NSAIDs can reduce or abolish bone pain. Morphine is only needed for severe bone pain where there is a continuous aching element to the pain (*see Bone Pain*).

Nerve pain is typically burning or stabbing, and can be extremely severe. It often responds only partially to morphine (which should always be tried first, as it will often decrease the pain to some extent) and tricyclics, steroids, anti-convulsants and occasionally nerve blocks or epidural drugs are also needed (*see Nerve pain*).

Secondary cancer pains include:

- Colicky pain
- Pleuritic pain
- Tenesmus
- Bladder spasms
- Central pain

Colicky pain typically comes and goes in waves (sometimes with nausea and dizziness) followed by pain-free intervals. It is most commonly seen in malignant intestinal obstruction, but can occasionally be renal or biliary. It does not respond to morphine, but can be controlled with anti-cholinergics, such as Buscopan 10-20mg QID orally, or 60 180mg over 24 hours by subcutaneous infusion. Ureteric pain can be continuous as well as colicy, and can be relieved by stents inserted at cystoscopy.

Pleuritic pain is a sharp chest pain on inspiration, usually due to infection or a pulmonary infarct following an embolus. Treatment options are paracetamol or indomethacin, antibiotics for pleurisy or an intra-pleural bupivacaine infusion via a catheter. Anti-coagulation may be appropriate occasionally for recurrent pulmonary infarcts (*see Deep Vein Thrombosis*).

Tenesmus is an unpleasant sensation of wanting to open the bowels, usually due to a rectal tumour or pelvic recurrence. Always exclude impacted faeces which can cause or worsen the symptom. It is caused by pressure on stretch receptors in the levator ani muscles, and can occur after AP resection of the rectum ("phantom rectum syndrome"). Treatment options include:

- Morphine
- Radiotherapy
- Laser
- Steroids
- Chlorpromazine

- Steroid enemas
- Local anaesthetic enema
- Lumbar sympathectomy

Tenesmus is usually only partially responsive to morphine. RT can help if there is a large cauliflower lesion, but is contra-indicated if there is vaginal involvement because of the risk of a recto-vaginal fistula. Laser therapy may also be considered for large inoperable lesions. High dose steroids can reduce peri-tumour oedema and swelling and may reduce tenesmus. Chlorpromazine is often quoted as helpful but there is no firm evidence in support of it. Some patients find steroid enemas (colifoam) daily or BD very helpful. Another treatment is bupivacaine (Marcaine) enemas which can give relief for several hours and sometimes after a few days of relief the pain is reduced in severity. Bilateral lumbar sympathetic neurolytic block can sometimes help to reduce tenesmus and should be considered if other treatments have not helped.

Bladder spasms cause severe intermittent suprapubic pains, sometimes radiating into the penis or perineum. If associated with urinary urgency it can be termed strangury. Suprapubic pain is usually due to mucosal irritation of the trigone, which may be referred to the urethra, and is commonest after radiotherapy for bladder cancer, or due to malignant infiltration of the bladder due to pelvic tumours. This pain can be severe and difficult to control. Exclude infection. If the patient has a catheter try reducing the balloon size to 2.5-5ml. Consider the following:

- Oxybutynin 5mg 8 hourly
- Instill 0.25% bupivacaine (20ml for 20 min)
- Subcutaneous Buscopan (60-180mg per 24 hours)
- Lumbar sympathetic block (bilateral)

Oxybutynin (Ditropan) is strongly anti-cholinergic and also has a calcium antagonist action, and can reduce bladder spasms, urgency or strangury.

Central pain is pain due to permanent neuronal changes that may have occured in the cortex, thalamus or spinal cord. An example is the phantom limb pain that can continue after the amputation of a painful ischaemic leg. It is rare in patients with cancer, but can occur following cord compression, when the lower half of the body has no sensation, yet severe pain can occur in the lower back and legs. This can only be explained by a central mechanism. It does not respond to morphine, but can respond very well to a combination of chlorpromazine (25-75mg 4 hourly) and amitriptyline (75-150mg at night).

Pelvic pain is discussed in the section on Pelvic recurrence.

Scar pain can occur after surgery, and is most commonly seen after thoracotomy. Post thoracotomy scar pain is due to traction on intercostal nerves. There is usually some sensory loss and an area of tenderness at the posterior end of the scar. It usually settles after 2 months. Persistent pain occurs in about 15% after thoracotomy and may be due to a nylon stitch, a traumatic neuroma or a recurrent pleural tumour. A sensitive trigger spot suggests a neuroma, which is relieved by an injection of local anaesthetic temporarily, and may require an intercostal nerve block or excision. CT scan may demonstrate recurrent tumour. A frozen shoulder can occur on the affected side. Post-mastectomy scar pain is due to damage to the intercosto-brachial nerve (cutaneous branch of T1,2) and occurs usually after post- operative complications. It causes burning pain in the posterior axilla, a tight sensation across chest, a tender spot (if a neuroma is present) and sometimes a frozen shoulder. Post-nephrectomy scar pain is due to damage to L1 and can cause a burning sensation (radiates to groin) and a sensation of heaviness in flank. Support from a corset can help if there is laxness of the muscles.

Pain threshold is a very useful concept when managing a difficult pain that cannot be completely controlled (usually a nerve pain). Pain control is then seen as having two components: Reduction of the pain and elevation of the pain threshold. The following help to raise the pain threshold:

- Control other symptoms
- Good quality sleep
- A feeling of security
- Psychological support
- Explanation
- Resolving emotional conflicts
- Relaxation\massage
- Diversional activities
- Treat anxiety or depression

It is common experience that mood and activity affect the appreciation of pain. Studies have shown that low self-esteem and low pain threshold are linked, and pain control can be improved by techniques to improve self-esteem. Exploration of the symbolic meaning of the pain in terms of the patient's life experience, culture, lifestyle and family interactions can improve the ability to cope. Avoid the expression "a low pain threshold". The pain threshold cannot be measured. If a patient complains a lot about pain, either they have pain or they have good reasons for complaining of pain. Excessive complaining may be due to "pain behaviour" rather than pain, when the patient gains something (such as attention) from complaining. A possible mechanism of action of emotional factors on pain is via the descending inhibitory pathways from the midbrain to the dorsal horn.

Pain Pathways. For many years pain was thought to be due to imbalance of humours, until 1664 when Descartes introduced the idea of a pain pathway running from the skin to the brain. We now know that the "pathway" is highly complex. The spinal cord is more like a tubular computer than an electric cable, and modulates the pain (the gate theory). The discovery in 1969 of descending inhibitory pathways (from the midbrain to the dorsal horn) is bringing us back to ideas of chronic pain being maintained by an imbalance of a variety of neuro-transmitters in the spinal cord and brain.

DIFFICULT PAINS – A CHECKLIST

Physical element?

- New pain?
- Morphine dose too low?
- Poor morphine absorbtion? (s\c infusion)
- Co-analgesic
- Radiotherapy
- Physical methods (skin traction, TENS)
- Epidural morphine
- Nerve block
- Chemotherapy
- Neurosurgery (very rarely)

Emotional element?

- Anger, guilt,
- Unresolved grief
- Fears (dying\pain recurring\going home)
- Anxiety state
- Depression
- Family non-communication

References:
Davidson P. Facilitating coping with cancer pain. Palliative Medicine 1988; 2: 107-114.
Bruera E. Intractable pain in patients with advanced head and neck tumours: a possible role of local infection. Cancer Treat Rep 1986; 70: 691-2.
Walker VA, Dicks B, Webb P. Pain assessment charts in the management of chronic cancer pain. Palliative Medicine 1987; 1: 111-116.

PANCREATIC CANCER

Pancreatic cancer causes around 6,800 deaths per year in the UK. It is difficult to diagnose and there is often a history of several months of pain (often causing depression) before the diagnosis is reached ("Could I have been cured?"). Diagnosis is based on biopsy either at laparotomy or by CT or ultrasound guided biopsy. The prognosis is very poor. 90% die within 1 year of diagnosis. Total pancreatectomy is possible for small tumours but the operative mortality is high and only 5% survive 5 years. Metastases occur to liver (and less commonly to lung, bone and brain). Radiotherapy is very disappointing.

Chemotherapy is disappointing and there is no standard regime for routine use. About 20% have some response to fluorouracil, but other regimes should be restricted to clinical trials.

Palliative surgery is helpful for cancers in the head of the pancreas (70%) which often cause obstructive jaundice and duodenal obstruction. Bypass surgery can prevent jaundice (cholecysto-jejunostomy) and duodenal obstruction (gastro-jejunostomy) but is not always technically possible. A coeliac plexus block should be performed at the same time.

Problems in advanced cancer of the pancreas include:

- Pain
- Ascites
- Obstructive jaundice (itch)
- Vomiting (duodenal obstruction)
- Steatorrhoea
- Ocsophageal varices (portal vein compression)

Pancreatic pain occurs in 85% and is continuous visceral pain that is classically epigastric, radiating into the back and partially relieved by leaning forwards. However it can also be referred to either hypochodrium or into the lower abdomen. A coeliac plexus block (CPB) should be considered early for pain that is not controlled by full doses of morphine. 90% get pain relief from a CPB (*see Nerve Blocks*).

Steatorrhoea (pale bulky stools) is due to malabsorbtion (due to blockage of the pancreatic duct and loss of pancreatic enzymes) causing diarrhoea that does not respond to anti-diarrhoeals but does respond to Pancreatic replacement (*see Diarrhoea*).

PARANOIA

Paranoia means a feeling of persecution, and may be "normal" or due to fear, confusion or depression.

"Normal" paranoia means that most patients are understandably pre-occupied with themselves, and in unfamiliar surroundings, such as a hospice, patients can misinterpret what they hear. In particular, be sure to include patients in any laughter.

Fear is common in advanced illness. Most patients have episodes of being frightened, but persistent denial can lead on to mild paranoia, when drugs or external factors are blamed for the illness. "This place is making me worse". Counselling and support focus on reality-testing ("If you were back at home in your own bed now, how do you think you would feel?"). A small dose of haloperidol, 3-5mg BD, may be helpful.

Confusion (due to brain metastases, infection, drugs) tends to cause disorientation, poor memory and agitation. Paranoia is also a common feature (*see Confusion*).

Severe depression can cause psychotic features, including paranoia, delusions and hallucinations (*see Depression*).

PELVIC RECURRENCE

Recurrence of pelvic tumours (cervix, rectum and bladder) causes similar clinical problems with:

- Pain
- Leg swelling (lymphoedema)
- Urinary symptoms
- Hydronephrosis
- Ureteric obstruction

Diagnosis of recurrent pelvic tumour is by CT scan, which may show a pre-sacral mass, enlarged nodes or hydronephrosis. Radiotherapy can be used to treat, and occasionally cure, patients who develop a recurrence after surgery. Radiotherapy or chemotherapy may shrink the tumour and control symptoms, and are indicated for patients who presented with advanced disease and have not yet had cancer treatment.

Pelvic pain may be unilateral iliac fossa pain, or hypogastric (from bladder or uterus) or rectal (with pressure on sitting down, or shooting pains or tenesmus) or in the low back (due to direct sacral invasion from a pre-sacral recurrence) or perineum, external genitalia or upper thighs. Pain radiating into the leg due to lumbo-sacral plexus infiltration is one of the most difficult pains to control (*see Nerve Pain*). Infiltration of the psoas muscle (which is rare) causes painful fixed flexion of the ipsilateral hip and pain in the anterior thigh (L1-3) which is worse when the hip is extended, and it can be confirmed by CT scan.

Leg lymphoedema is usually unilateral, but can become bilateral. Compression therapy helps. Radiotherapy may be considered where it has not already been given (*see Lymphoedema*).

Urinary problems start as hesitancy due to nerve damage, and the patient may have to force the flow and assist by suprapubic pressure.

Ureteric obstruction causes unilateral hydronephrosis, seen on CT scan (or it may be suspected from renal pain or a rising creatinine). It is a bad prognostic sign which indicates increasing renal damage. Ureteric obstruction in a relatively fit patient may be an indication for surgery with:

- Ureteric stents
- Ureteric bypass
- Percutaneous nephrostomy
- Permanent nephrostomy

Bilateral ureteric obstruction is usually seen as a terminal event. However, surgery is justified if the prognosis seems reasonable (deterioration over months rather than weeks) or if further treatment is possible or if a benign radiation stricture cannot be excluded or if the patient insists on surgery. Surgical relief of bilateral obstruction (by stenting or nephrostomy) needs to be carefully considered, (ideally by the informed and supported patient and family) because a peaceful death from uraemia may be exchanged for a prolonged death with increasing pain and discharge from the tumour.

Ureteric stent can be inserted by a urologist. The orifice of the ureter may have to be exposed by endoscopic resection of tumour. A catheter is introduced into the ureter under Xray control, then a guide-wire and then the self-retaining stent.

Ureteric by-pass surgery may be possible. This may involve ureteric implant into the colon, or an ileal conduit.

Percutaneous nephrostomy is temporary and can be performed quickly and a more permanent nephrostomy performed later if it is still appropriate.

Fistulas can occur in far-advanced pelvic disease and may be:

- Vesico-vaginal (continuous dribbling)
- Recto-vaginal (continuous faecal leak)
- Recto-vesical (urine infection and debris)

Palliative surgery (ileal diversion or colostomy) should be considered whenever possible for these distressing symptoms. Explanation and support can reduce guilt and isolation.

Discharge from the tumour may be profuse and foul smelling. Metronidazole can reduce smell, tranexamic acid can control bleeding. Change dressings regularly.

Radiation damage or recurrent tumour? This question arises after treatment of cancer of the cervix when small bowel damage, (with stenosis and obstruction) or fistulas (from the rectum or bladder into the vagina) occur. The patient may require bowel resections, colostomy or urinary diversion, (and sometimes all three). CT scan (even with guided biopsy) may not be able to distinguish areas of radiation fibrosis from recurrent cancer. If time passes and the patient's condition remains stable, the picture of radiation damage without recurrence becomes apparent.

PLEURAL EFFUSION

Pleural effusion means fluid in the pleural cavity. It occurs in 5% of hospice patients. It is caused by cancers of the bronchus and breast and occasionally other tumours (mesothelioma, ovary, lymphoma).

Mechanism: malignant infiltration of the pleura and reduced circulation and reabsorbtion of pleural fluid (500cc per day) that serves to lubricate the pleural surfaces. Malignant effusions are usually urine-coloured, but may be blood-stained or chylous (milky white) due to lymph leaking from the thoracic duct). N.B. The underlying lung may be normal.

Prognosis. A malignant pleural effusion is usually a feature of far-advanced disease, but some patients can survive for many months, especially in breast cancer and mesothelioma.

Symptoms of a pleural effusion are dyspnoea, cough and pleuritic pains, but if the fluid accumulates slowly, it may cause no symptoms. Signs are absent breath sounds and dullness to percussion.

Chest Xray shows a basal opacity and a surface meniscus laterally. If there is doubt whether the opacity is an effusion, or pleural thickening or basal consolidation, a lateral decubitus Xray or ultrasound scan can confirm fluid.

Management options for pleural effusion include:

- Chemotherapy
- Morphine
- Pleural aspiration
- Sclerosants
- Pleurectomy
- Antibody-guided irradiation

Chemotherapy may control an effusion in cancer of the breast or in small cell cancer of the lung. Radiotherapy is not helpful (except in lymphoma).

Morphine can control cough and dyspnoea and may be the best treatment in advanced disease, if the effusion is recurring rapidly or if it is causing only mild symptoms (*see Morphine*).

Pleural aspiration is a simple outpatient procedure. It is indicated to relieve dyspnoea. The fluid tends to re- accumulate over 1-4 weeks, when the procedure can easily be repeated. If the patient is on warfarin in must be stopped or reversed with vitamin K (*see Bleeding*) before the procedure (see below).

Sclerosants. If an effusion recurs rapidly, then a sclerosant can be used to try to slow down the re-accumulation of fluid. It is most effective if it is instilled after the effusion is drained to dryness.

Bleomycin (1.25mg per kg, usually 90mg, but not exceeding 40mg in the frail or elderly) will control the effusion for about 1 month in 70% of cases. 100mg hydrocortisone given first reduces the incidence of fever and pain due to pleural reaction. After instillation the patient is placed in various positions to promote a diffuse pleural response. Bleomycin is the most suitable of the many sclerosants that have been used (including tetracycline, quinacrine, nitrogen mustard, adriamycin, mitoxantrone, interferon, talc and

Corynebacterium parvum). There have been few randomized trials comparing these agents.

Pleurectomy is the definitive surgical treatment, and effectively controls a pleural effusion in 90% of cases, but the post-operative mortality is 10%.

Antibody-guided irradiation may come to have a place in treatment. In one study 10 out of 13 effusions (7 pleural, 3 pericardial) responded completely with no fluid re- accumulation for 3-18 months. (Reference: Pectasides D *et al*. Antibody-guided irradiation fo malignant pleural and pericardial effusions. Br J Cancer (1986); 53: 727-732)

Procedure of pleural aspiration. Use a set with a small- bore needle, since a wide-bore needle used for pleural biopsies is not necessary. Attach the plastic tubing to the needle first, then the 3-way tap, then the 50cc syringe (this arrangement of the tubing allows the operator to move the syringe about, without moving the needle). The operator sits behind the patient. The patient leans forward onto some pillows and rests his head on his folded arms. Use bupivacaine (Marcain) 0.25%, 10ml, to numb the skin. N.B. wait a few minutes for skin numbness to occur.

The puncture site is usually laterally in the sixth intercostal space or 1 or 2 spaces below the upper border of the dullness (a common mistake is to aim too low, at the level of the costo-phrenic angle of pleura. Insert the needle on top of a rib, (to avoid the neurovascular bundle). An alternative to a 3-way tap is a simple method of using a 14 G venous cannula connected to a standard surgical drainage bottle (Redivac), which exerts only 10cm H2O negative pressure and stops as it fills up, after 250-500cc. Aim to remove about 0.5-1.5 litres of fluid.

Problems are uncommon. If the fluid is removed too quickly or in too great a quantity it can cause pulmonary oedema in the expanding lung (very rare). If fluid is difficult to obtain it may be loculated (which can be seen on ultrasound) or the needle may be too low (if it is in the diaphragm the pleura feels stiff and the needle moves widely with respiration) – replace the needle a bit higher. If the fluid becomes harder to draw into the syringe, it may be due to the inability of the underlying lung to re-expand, (especially if the effusion is long-standing) with increasing negative intrapleural pressure. Stop if there is pain, coughing or dizziness, (mediastinal shift) which can be relieved by letting air into the pleural space.

The main risk is a large pneumothorax (air in the pleural space) either by a tear in the visceral pleura or via the chest wall. The risk is much less when tapping a large effusion. Chest Xray shows a lung edge with no vascular markings lateral to it. If a pneumothorax causes dyspnoea or pain it must be treated by the insertion of an intercostal drain and underwater seal to remove the air.

PRESCRIBING

Good prescribing is a skill, and makes the difference between poor and excellent symptom control. Knowledge is required of correct drugs, correct doses, correct route and correct frequency, being aware of:

- Contra-indications
- Drug interactions
- Side-effects
- Allergies

Twice daily oral dosage had the same compliance rate as once daily dosage, in one study, of 70-75%, and may be the optimum method of prescribing, because loss of therapeutic benefit is less after a missed dose than for once a day medication.

The principles of good prescribing are to monitor the effects of treatment and adjust the doses for optimum effect. It is a good rule to make one drug change at a time, as far as possible. Other important aspects are:

- Explain all changes
- Use a drug card
- Explain to relatives
- Stop drugs that have not helped
- Stop unnecessary drugs (e.g. hypotensives)

Preferences for particular medicines, likes and dislikes should be recorded on the drug chart. This improves compliance. Allergies must be carefully noted on the drug chart as well as the medical record.

A drug card is an essential and simple tool for outpatient prescribing. It is a grid, with drugs listed down the lefthand column, times to be taken (usually 9,1,5,9) across the top of the card and the purpose for the drugs down the righthand column. It should be written with the patient and relatives – time invested at this stage greatly improves compliance and improves symptom control. The patient should bring it to all appointments, which also improves communication between doctors.

Compliance aids such as daily or weekly pill dispensers, with compartments for the pills to be taken at each meal time can be helpful. They can be pre-loaded by carers for patients who are living alone but finding it difficult to cope with all the medication. Mistakes can still be made by the patient who gets confused. Bottle top adaptors (to allow accurate dispensing of liquid medication) can be helpful.

Inpatient prescribing offers opportunities (not always taken) to control symptoms by carefully monitoring the effects of drugs and doses. The principles are:

- Use drug chart correctly
- Liaise with pharmacist
- PRN drugs for nurse's use
- Explain all changes (patient and relatives)
- Simplify regime before discharge
- Write drug card before discharge

The ward pharmacist should be invited to attend some ward rounds, for doctors and pharmacists to communicate about the drugs being prescribed.

PRN drugs are given as required (Pro Re Nata means when the need arises) and are particularly important in the context of symptom control, because they empower the nurses to keep the patient comfortable if minor symptoms such as headache occur, or if the patient's condition suddenly deteriorates. Most hospice inpatients routinely have the following drugs written up on the PRN part of the drug chart:

- Paracetamol (1g 4 hourly) – headaches
- IM diamorphine, (half the oral dose 4 hourly)
- IM chlorpromazine (25-50mg 4 hourly)
- IM hyoscine (0.4mg 4 hourly)
- Stesolid 10mg PR (if risk of seizures)

PRN analgesics for chronic pain are generally avoided. In the context of the control of cancer pain PRN can stand for Pain Relief Non-existent.

The route of administration of drugs sometimes needs to be carefully considered. Options include:

- Oral
- Rectal
- Sublingual
- Buccal
- Transdermal
- Subcutaneous
- Inhaled
- IM
- IV

IV drugs are rarely needed in symptom control, one exception being IV midazolam, which can be useful to control severe terminal dyspnoea and panic. IV diamorphine is avoided because it is the only route by which tolerance develops (*see Morphine*).

The transdermal route can be used for drugs with a low molecular weight, where only a few mg are needed per day, and is used for hyoscine, nitrates, clonidine and oestradiol. Fentanyl, a potent opioid, can be given transdermally, although its high lipid solubility means the plasma levels rise only slowly at first. It may come to have a place in the terminal phase, as an alternative to IM injections or SC infusion in the home care setting.

PRESSURE SORES

Pressure sores are areas of skin damage caused by capillary pressure and ischaemia. Friction also causes skin damage (lifting, turning). The main sites occur over bony prominences – sacrum, hip, heel, ankle and elbow. 2 hours of unrelieved pressure above 30 mm Hg can cause cell death. The effects of pressure and pressure relief on capillary function remains poorly understood.

CLASSIFICATION OF PRESSURE SORES BY COLOUR		
Pressure sore	Healing time (if pressure relieved)	Possible dressing
1. Early Redness	2 days	Semi- permeable
2. Red + ulcers	1-2 weeks	Hydrocolloid
3. Yellow + exudate	weeks	Foam
4. Black necrotic	weeks	Hydrogel
5. Cavity	months	Alginate ribbon

Risk factors for developing pressure sores can be assessed by various scores, (e.g. Waterlow) the main factors being;

- Age
- Weight
- Skin condition (oedema, redness)
- Continence
- Mobility
- Nutrition
- Sensory loss\paraplegia
- Steroids\cytotoxics

Principles of treating pressure sores include:

- Relieve pressure
- Improve mobility
- Reduce friction damage
- Moist wound healing (modern dressings)
- Remove slough (delays healing)
- Avoid topical antiseptics\antibiotics

Healing occurs if the pressure sore is relieved of pressure. Sores cannot and need not be made sterile, but heal better with warmth and moisture. Colonization with moderate numbers of pathogenic bacteria does <u>not</u> delay healing.

Slough (a yellow layer of fibrin, pus and dead tissue) should be removed. It will delay healing because it contains proteolytic enzymes and it predisposes to infection. Early slough can often be removed with warm saline.

Antiseptics are only needed for dirty or infected sores. Chlorhexidine 0.05% is recommended as the most suitable antiseptic. Healing is delayed by using cold fluids (which slow healing) and strong antiseptics (especially chlorine-based solutions, such as Eusol or hypochlorite) which damage fibroblasts and delay granulation.

Infection that is more than superficial and causing surrounding cellulitis, will delay healing and requires an oral antibiotic. Take a swab and start flucloxacillin (for staphylococci) and metronidazole (for anaerobes) until the results of culture and sensitivities are available.

Topical antibiotics have no advantages over antiseptics and can cause contact dermatitis, but there are 2 exceptions: Metronidazole gel 0.8% (Metrotop) will control smell very effectively (*see Smell*) and silver sulphadiazine (Flamazine cream) will prevent infection in burns.

N.B. Avoid massage around the sore area, which can increase skin damage.

Reddened areas can be protected with a semi-permeable film (Opsite, Tegaderm, Bioclusive) to reduce the likelihood of ulceration and to speed healing. If redness blanches on touch it suggests the capillaries are still intact and healing will occur in a few hours if pressure is relieved. Non-blanching redness takes 48 hours of pressure relief to heal.

Yellow exudate forms once there is skin ulceration. It can be absorbed with a hydrocolloid, hydrogel, alginate, or foam dressing – each has its advocates. All of them are designed to promote moist wound healing and granulation (*see Dressings*).

Slough should be removed as it inhibits healing due to proteolytic enzymes. Debris will float if softened, so moist (but not soggy conditions) should be maintained. Superficial slough may be removed by bathing or saline irrigation under pressure. Dry slough can be removed with hydrogel dressings, or if stubborn, desloughing agents such as Aserbine (chemical) or streptokinase (biological). Thick slough can be painlessly removed with a scalpel.

Cavities need to be packed loosely with tulle dressings or Sorbsan ribbon (which is bio-degradable, so strands left behind are simply absorbed). These allow granulation (and prevent premature closure and abscess formation). Avoid dry gauze, tight packing and antiseptics like hypochlorite, Eusol or povidone iodine, because they damage new granulation tissue and slow healing. Sialastic foam plugs are useful in the community as they need changing less frequently. New plugs need to be made (by pouring the liquid into the cavity, which sets into the foam) as the cavity heals and gets smaller.

Pressure relief is best achieved by improving the patient's mobility, but when this is not possible, the following are helpful:

- Heel and elbow pads (Spenco, sheepskin)
- Fibre mattress (e.g. Spenco)
- Foam mattress (e.g. Propad)

- Pegasus bi-wave mattress
- Pegasus air wave mattress
- Specialized beds

Fibre mattresses (Spenco) pads are useful, and reduce shearing forces, but after washing the mattress covers can become lumpy and uncomfortable.

Foam mattresses (Pro-pad) that are placed on top of a normal mattress are very comfortable and should ideally be used for all bedbound patients. A waterproof cover is available for incontinent patients.

The Pegasus biwave mattress is placed on top of an ordinary bed. It reduces skin pressure by deflation and re-inflation of air cells.

The Pegasus airwave mattress replaces the normal mattress, and is used for weak patients, and reduces the need to turn the patient. There is zero pressure on the skin for 30% of the time in each 7 minute cycle.

Specialized beds "suspend" the patient on air sacs (Mediscus) or microspheres (Clinitron). They are very expensive. See the section on Equipment for useful addresses.

Physiotherapy. To improve a patient's mobility and independence is the best way to prevent or heal pressure sores. Weak patients need careful lifting and moving to avoid friction and shearing forces on the skin, which tear capillaries. Bedbound patients need 2 hourly turning. Physical methods are sometimes tried, to promote granulation tissue, including ice therapy, ultraviolet light, ultrasound, ionized water vapour, pulsed high frequency energy and laser.

Plastic surgery (skin grafts, muscle flaps) may be needed for deep tissue damage, but this is rarely seen in terminal illness, and is mainly seen in longterm disabled patients, due to arterial compression, resulting in skin damage which is full thickness from the start.

In dying patients comfort is the priority, rather than healing. A Pegasus mattress increases patient comfort. An ordinary barrier cream (such as zinc and castor oil) covered with an a dry dressing will sooth the sore and prevent friction.

Reference:
Gilcrest B, Corner J. Pressure sores: prevention and management – a nursing perspective. Palliative Medicine 1989; 3: 257-261.

PROSTATIC CANCER

Prostatic cancer causes around 8000 deaths per year in the UK. It usually presents with urinary hesitancy or pains from bone metastases. 50% of patients already have bone metastases at presentation, when the median survival is only 3 years (although 10% survive 10 years). Diagnosis is strongly suspected from a raised serum acid phosphatase and is confirmed by biopsy (usually trans-rectal). Most tumours are well-differentiated adenocarcinomas.

Localized disease with no metastases may be treated with curative radiotherapy, 6000 cGy over 6 weeks, (which may cause some severe proctitis) but 30% will go on to develop previously undetected metastases within 2 years. Prostatectomy is becoming popular in the US for younger patients, where new techniques are reducing the post- operative complications of impotence, stricture or incontinence. Older patients with a small tumour can remain asymptomatic for years (and often have a higher risk of dying from cardiovascular disease than their tumour), and palliative management is usually advised for older patients (TURP and hormone therapy if symptoms develop, with palliative radiotherapy for any bone pain).

Metastases commonly occur to bone and pelvic lymph nodes, and less commonly to liver and lung. Radiotherapy or Strontium 89 may be used for bone pain (*see Bone pain*). Chemotherapy has no role in cancer of the prostate.

Hormone therapy produces a response in 80% and will improve symptoms for some months. However, early hormone manipulation (by castration or anti-androgens) does not prolong survival and it can be reasonable to delay treatment until symptoms occur, since the best response occurs when hormone manipulation is first started (*see Hormone Therapy*).

Problems of advanced cancer of the prostate include:

- Bone pains
- Anaemia
- Urinary hesitancy
- Rectal narrowing
- Lymphoedema of the leg(s)
- Ulcerated inguinal nodes

Urinary hesitancy is often not a problem, but if it recurs then TURP can be repeated or a prostatic stent inserted.

Rectal stenosis is rarely complete and can be managed with softening agents.

PSYCHOLOGICAL THERAPY

Adjuvant psychological therapy (APT) is a programme of support for cancer patients being developed at the Royal Marsden Hospital. It is a brief problem-focused cognitive and behavioural programme of weekly sessions of 1 hour, for 4-8 weeks, designed to focus on the personal meaning of cancer to the individual and on coping strategies, i.e. what they think and do to reduce the threat imposed by the cancer. Therapy is directed at the current problems as defined jointly with the therapist. APT focuses on challenging negative thinking, developing realistic goals, expressing strong emotions, improving communications with a partner and relaxation.

Cognitive techniques include identifying personal strengths, raising self-esteem, reducing feelings of helplessness, promoting a fighting spirit, identifying negative automatic thoughts and challenging negative automatic thoughts. Behavioural techniques include using imagination and role play to reduce the stress of impending events, encouraging activities that give a sense of pleasure in order to regain a feeling of control, encouraging ventilation of feelings, encouraging open communication with partner and relaxation techniques to overcome episodes of anxiety (*see Further reading*).

A prospective randomized controlled trial of this therapy has been reported in 72 cancer patients (with a life expectancy of at least 12 months) who had psychological disorders lasting more than 4 weeks from the time of diagnosis or news of recurrence (to exclude acute stress reactions). Patients randomized to receive therapy (median 5 treatments) showed a significant reduction in anxiety, falling from 46% of the patients originally to 20% at 8 weeks and 20% at 4 months, with little change in controls. Depression also fell from 40% to 13% at 8 weeks and 18% at 4 months, with little change in controls. After treatment the Mental Adjustment to Cancer Scale showed significantly higher scores for fighting spirit and significantly lower scores for helplessness, anxious pre-occupation and fatalism.

Reference:
Greer S, Moorey S *et al.* Adjuvant psychological therapy for patients with cancer: a prospective randomized trial. Br Med J 1992; 304: 675-80.

Psychological defenses are ways of coping with the threat of cancer. It is more useful to look at ways of coping than to apply psychiatric labels. Ways of coping can be classified as:

- Denial
- Fatalism
- Helpless and hopeless
- Anxious pre-occupation
- Fighting spirit
- Active acceptance

Defensive denial, caused by fear, is discussed in the section on anxiety. Defensive denial is different to the deliberate non-attention that may be encouraged as a way of coping, once the necessary adjustments have been made, and which is completely lacking in patients with *anxious pre-occupation. Fatalism* involves a passive acceptance ("I'll leave it all in your hands doctor"). APT aims to induce a *fighting spirit,* which usually implies a non-acceptance of dying. However, *active acceptance*, resulting from a spiritual adjustment, is also a good way of coping for some.

Negative thinking is self-defeating. It under-estimates coping abilities and the help available from others and over-estimates the probability and severity of problems. It includes:

- Negative predictions
- Overgeneralizations
- Disasterization ("everything's gone wrong")
- Self-labelling
- Self-blame
- Mind-reading (negative assumptions)

THE RESULTS OF
CHALLENGING NEGATIVE THINKING

Negative Thinking	Positive Re-framing by the patient (not the therapist)
I'm useless	I'm not as strong as I was and need to adjust my lifestyle.
We're always arguing now	We had a disagreement because of the pressure we've both been under.
I may as well be dead.	The disease can't be cured, but I may have months of useful life left.
Life is pointless.	Life has changed, but there are still things that I can enjoy.
My family don't care about me.	I sometimes wished my family showed more affection, but when they do I often tell them not to make a fuss.
I can't even do the gardening now	I feel guilty about leaving things to others, forgetting that I am ill.

Cognitive therapy is based on the assumption that a person can learn to change habitual negative thinking and thereby reduce their own distress. Negative thinking can be challenged using the ABC approach. A = Attitudes or thoughts that are causing the unpleasant feelings, which must first be identified, B = Belief that the attitude is based on, and C = Challenge to that belief. Challenging a person's thinking is both possible and helpful. To quote Shakespeare (Hamlet, act 2, scene 2, line 254) "... for there is nothing either good or bad but thinking makes it so". Some results of challenging and re-framing thinking are given in the table, but it is important to understand that the positive thinking is arrived at by the patient after a period of time, and cannot simply be imposed by a therapist. Examples of ways of challenging a thought might be:

- Is it true?
- What's the evidence?
- Are there alternative ways of looking at it?
- If true, is it really that bad?

Patients who cope well tend to be those who show some of the following characteristics. They try to adjust to their illness and dependency, participate in their care, seek information, and try to be optimistic. They retain some control over their life, face up to fears (rather than denying fears), and have realistic short-term goals. Socially, they maintain some interest in events, sort out their affairs, communicate with relatives and deal with unfinished emotional business. Most importantly, they search for some sense of purpose or meaning in what is happening to them (*see Spiritual support*).

A diary of mood, thoughts and activities can help some patients identify problems that can be tackled and can reduce feelings of helplessness. The diary has 4 columns for date and time, mood (simply scored 1-10), thoughts recorded in some detail and activity at the time (e.g. TV, crossword, phone call home, eating lunch etc.). Associations may become apparent between certain activities and negative thinking, and such a diary can provide a method of containing very strong or destructive emotions.

Reference:
Jones K, Johnston M, Speck P. Despair felt by the patient and the professional carer: a case study of the use of cognitive behavioural methods. Palliative Medicine 1989; 3: 39-46.

Further reading:
Moorey S, Greer S. Psychological therapy for patient's with cancer. Heinemann Medical Books, 1989.

RADIOTHERAPY

50% of cancer patients require radiotherapy at some stage, and half of all treatments are palliative.

Curative Radiotherapy is high dose ("radical") radiotherapy, which aims to deliver radiation to the limits of tissue tolerance, in order to attempt eradication of the tumour. Once a radical dose has been given, no further radiotherapy can usually be given to that area again. High dose radiotherapy is used as sole treatment for primary tumours of the larynx, head and neck, cervix, seminoma, early lymphomas, early lung, early prostate, anus, thyroid and advanced bladder. RT is is used with surgery in the primary treatment of cancers of breast, rectum, advanced head and neck and sarcomas.

Fractionation of the dose damages malignant cells more than normal cells, since malignant cells recover more slowly between fractions. It also reduces side-effects. Total dose, number of fractions, dose per fraction and total length of treatment all affect the amount of tissue damage, e.g. a single dose of 10 Gy has a much bigger effect than 10 daily doses of 1 Gy.

CHART is a new approach to fractionation, and trials are in progress for cancers of the head and neck and for non-small cell lung cancers. CHART means continuous hyperfractionated accelerated radiation therapy, the principle being to give the RT as quickly as possible to kill rapidly dividing cells. Instead of daily fractions for 6 weeks, the total dose is given in 6 hourly fractions for 12 consecutive days.

Radio-sensitivity of tumours varies. For example to control a 2cm tumour requires about 25 Gy if it is a seminoma, 40 Gy for a lymphoma, and 60 Gy for a squamous cancer, and doses over 70 Gy will not control a similar sized astrocytoma. Resistance to radiation may be due to rapid cell proliferation and to overcome this a new approach is being tried to give RT fractions through the day, as rapidly as possible, which is called continuous hyperfractionated accelerated radiotherapy (CHART).

Planning of treatment on a simulator is needed to decide on the size of the field to be treated (to include malignant nodes for example) and to compute the doses required. Multifield techniques and megavoltage machines allow high doses to be delivered to deep tumours without damage to normal tissues.

Palliative radiotherapy is relatively low dose radiotherapy, intended to control symptoms. It can reduce tumour bulk and relieve symptoms, but does not significantly eradicate cancer cells. The dose varies from 8 Gy in a single dose for bone pain in a long bone, to 20Gy over 4 days for a lung tumour, to 40 Gy over 4 weeks to shrink a tumour of the head and neck or pelvis. Palliative RT is used for:

- Bone pain
- To shrink nodes
- To relieve obstruction (SVC, bronchus, oesophagus)
- To control cutaneous spread
- To control haemorrhage
- Spinal cord compression
- Brain metastases

Palliative RT is not effective for ascites or pleural effusions or peritoneal tumours, and nerve plexus damage is rarely reversed.

Hypofractionation has been unpopular amongst radiotherapists, who are rightly concerned to minimize side-effects of therapy. However, for patients with a short prognosis a single treatment of 8Gy, regardless of volume, can be very effective palliative treatment for some symptoms, and can be repeated after a week if necessary.

Radical or Palliative? Patients are sometimes confused by their palliative treatment ("If the doctors knew I had cancer cells in my body, why didn't they treat me sooner"). The difference between radical, high dose, curative radiotherapy, and palliative low dose radiotherapy often needs explaining. Radical radiotherapy aims to cure, and the highest dose that the body can tolerate is given in the hope of killing all the cancer cells. Side-effects are therefore more common. Palliative doses are lower and aim to control symptoms rather than cure.

Side-effects of palliative RT include:

- Nausea (RT to abdomen, mediastinum)
- Reversible hair loss (RT to brain)
- Skin reaction

Skin reactions occurs at the site of RT. It is more common with orthovoltage machines, although mega-voltage machines can cause a skin reaction on the contra-lateral side of the body, where the X-rays exit the body. Redness and soreness begins 2-3 weeks after the first treatment and lasts 2-3 weeks after the last treatment. Dry desquamation, skin oedema and moist desquamation can all occur before healing occurs. Continued RT on moist desquamation can produce severe skin necrosis. For 2-3 weeks after RT the patient is usually advised to wear soft cotton clothes and to avoid:

- Wetting the skin
- Shaving the skin
- Perfumed soaps or lotions
- Strong sunlight

Soreness of the skin can be treated with 1% hydrocortisone cream.

Reference:
Horwich A. Radiotherapy Update. Br Med J 1992; 304: 1554-1557.

RECTAL CANCER

Rectal cancer causes around 6500 deaths per year in the UK. It typically presents with altered bowel habit (diarrhoea, mucus, blood) or tenesmus. 50% are palpable on rectal examination. Diagnosis is by sigmoidoscopy and barium enema. Most patients present with advanced disease. At presentation only 60% are operable, and only 40% of these patients are cured. If recurrence occurs within 2 years of surgery, prognosis is usually less than 12 months. Anterior resection, (with re-anastomosis of the bowel) is performed if the cancer is high, but low-lying cancers require A.P.

(abdomino-perineal) excision and permanent colostomy, which leaves male patients impotent. Post-operative radiotherapy is often given to reduce the risk of pelvic or sacral curve recurrence.

Recurrence after re-anastomosis causes rectal discharge and bleeding, or pain. Difficulty sitting down is pathognomonic of recurrence. Recurrence following AP resection, causes perineal skin nodules, pelvic pain, urinary symptoms or PV bleeding and CT scan often shows a pre-sacral mass. Metastases commonly occur to the liver (and later to lung, bone or brain). Most patients with metastases die within 1 year.

Chemotherapy can be considered for reasonably strong patients with symptoms. Fluorouracil with folinic acid gives the best response rates of around 30%. Higher doses give better response but with more toxicity (nausea, hair loss). it is usually given monthly for 4-6 months if there is a response. Hepatic artery infusion of drugs has no advantages and is a research tool. Solitary metastases in liver or lung can be resected, when post-operative survival for 5 years has been described.

Problems in advanced cancer of the rectum include:

- Nerve pain in the leg
- Lymphoedema of the leg
- Tenesmus
- Rectal discharge
- Perineal cavitation

In a study of 19 patients with pre-sacral recurrence the median survival was 11 months (range 1-39 months). 15 had RT for pain control, with significant improvement at first, but only for a median of 5 months. 10 patients required permanent catheterization and 5 had significant leg weakness (Reference: Palliative Medicine 1992; 6: 167-8).

See also Pelvic Recurrence.

REHABILITATION

Rehabilitation can be defined as enabling a person to achieve their maximum potential for living. Control of physical symptoms often allows rehabilitation to take place. Physical and mental rehabilitation go hand in hand. There has often been a loss of confidence, when rehabilitation will be resisted until confidence has been restored.

3 distinct situations can be usefully distinguished.

- Impairment (e.g. weak legs)
- Disability (e.g. difficulty walking)
- Handicap (e.g. inability to go shopping)

An impairment may be a much greater handicap for one person that another.

Physical deterioration is not always due to progression of the underlying disease, and may be reversible, e.g.

- Error with medication
- Poor sleep
- Stopping steroids
- Treatable infection
- Blocked shunt
- Depression
- Loss of confidence due to a fall

A step-by-step approach is necessary. To get a bedbound patient home again, the following steps are often needed:

1. Self-care (nursing)
2. Mobility (physiotherapy)
3. Living skills (O.T.)
4. Home assessment
5. Trial at home
6. Day care

1 Self-care includes washing, feeding, toileting and dressing and is the first step towards physical rehabilitation. Nursing care can actually reduce a patient's ability to be self-caring, and the nursing team may need a plan of graded reduction of nursing support.

2 Mobility (transfering, walking, stairs) can usually be improved by skilful physiotherapy, and using the appropriate aids (walking stick, frames) or teaching carers about lifting and transfering.

3. Living skills can be assessed as an inpatient by the O.T. and will usually involve preparing food and cooking.

4. Home assessment by the O.T. alone or with the patient, can enable aids and adaptions to be ordered in time for discharge home.

5. A Trial period at home of a few hours or a day and night, is a good way of increasing the confidence of the patient and family – it needs careful planning and may be best either at the week-end or during the week. The knowledge that an inpatient bed will be available if there are any crises often gives the patient and the family the confidence to try and make the transition home.

6. Day Care can encourage discharge home, by providing ongoing support to patient and carers.

Family carers need careful explanation of the plan, opportunities to express worries, and reassurance of ongoing support. This increases the liklihood of successful rehabilitation and discharge home of the patient.

Wheelchair mobility may be the aim if the patient is paraplegic or very weak. The chair and chair cushion need to selected after an assessment by the O.T. of the patient's requirements and home layout. There are 66 wheelchairs available from the DHS, The main ones are 9L (small rear wheel for pushing), 8L (large rear wheel for self-propelling) and 8BL (narrow version of 8L). Model 8 chairs have detachable foot-rests and arm rests for transfering.

Occupational therapy (OT) focuses on social rehabilitation which includes:

- Personal appearance
- Personal well-being
- Work (productive use of time)
- Recreation (relaxation, amusement, self-expression)
- Conversation
- Arts, crafts, poetry, music

Skillful OT aims to adapt activities to the appropriate level of energy and dependence. Engaging in familiar activities, or even learning new skills, reduces frustration and increases self-esteem. Creating or producing is "doing" as opposed to "being done to" and can restore a sense of purpose.

RENAL CANCER

Renal cancer (hypernephroma) causes around 2700 deaths per year in the UK. It is an adenocarcinoma (arising from tubular epithelium). 7% occur in the renal pelvis and are urothelial tumours, and may be associated with other tumours in the ureter and bladder. It usually presents as painless haematuria, (sometimes with pain, a lump, or a bone metastasis).

Treatment is surgical. Radical nephrectomy and post-operative RT cures 50-70% of localized disease. Resection of the primary tumour together with a solitary metastasis (bone, brain, liver) can occasionally produce a long disease-free interval. Locally advanced disease may involve the abdominal wall or diaphragm, and patients rarely survive more than 18 months. Radiotherapy can delay progression of advanced disease or control renal bleeding.

Metastases occur to bone (40%) lung (cannonball shadows), brain, liver and skin.

Chemotherapy has a low response rate of around 20% and there is no established place for chemotherapy. Medroxyprogesterone is sometimes given, and about 5% respond. Alpha interferon is also licensed for use in renal cancers, but as yet its role is uncertain.

Problems in advanced cancer of the kidney include:

- IVC Thrombosis
- Haematuria
- Rare features

IVC Thrombosis is due to spread of tumour along the renal vein. This can cause bilateral leg oedema, and can also block the hepatic veins causing jaundice and ascites (Budd-Chiari syndrome). Anticoagulation can improve these problems, and eventually collateral veins on the abdominal wall open up and the symptoms can then resolve.

Haematuria due to renal tumours can be controlled by RT or embolization (*see Bleeding*).

Rare features of this tumour are fevers, hypertension, polycythaemia and hypercalcaemia and heart failure due to A-V malformations in the tumour.

SARCOMAS

Soft tissue sarcomas cause around 600 deaths per year in the UK. They are malignant tumours of connective tissue, most commonly in fat (liposarcoma) or muscle (leiomyosarcoma). They usually present as a painless lump, and can reach an enormous size if not excised. Diagnosis is by CT scan. It is treated by wide local excision or amputation. Sarcomas are relatively resistant to radiotherapy and chemotherapy. Recurrence may occur in nodes, liver or lungs, when the median survival is only 12 months, although if a solitary metastasis in the lung can be excised, 25% survive 5 years. Recurrent disease grows more rapidly than the original tumour ("downgrading").

Osteosarcomas are rare primary malignant tumours of bone, most commonly affecting the age group of 10-20 years. There are about 150 new cases per year in the UK. They present with pain and swelling, most commonly around the knee. Treatment used to be by amputation, but now involves pre-operative chemotherapy and specialized surgery to remove affected bone and insert large internal prostheses, following which 50-70% can survive 3 years. Bone pain from recurrent disease responds to radiotherapy. Metastases usually affect the lungs, and a single pulmonary metastasis can be resected.

SEIZURES

A seizure (convulsion, epileptic fit) is an abnormal electrical discharge in the brain. Siezures only occur in about 1% of hospice patients.

Causes of seizures: Primary and secondary brain tumours can cause seizures. About 20% of patients with known brain metastases have some kind of seizure.

Generalized seizures cause loss of consciousness, spasms (tonic phase), jerking movements (clonic phase) then usually a period of sleep.

Focal seizures cause uncontrollable jerking of the face, arm or leg and are more frightening because the patient is conscious. They can become generalized, with loss of consciousness.

Emergency treatment of seizures is the same for generalized and focal siezures, with rectal diazepam.

Diazepam enema (Stesolid) 10mg comes with a rectal applicator and works as quickly as the IV route. It can be repeated for a prolonged convulsion, up to 40mg if necessary, with little risk of respiratory depression occuring. IV diazepam (diazemuls) 5-10mg is only needed occasionally if the rectal route is ineffective.

Anti-convulsants are given to prevent recurrence. Phenytoin (Epanutin), 200-400mg nocte, is an effective anti-convulsant. It takes 4-7 days to reach therapeutic levels; if quick control is needed an IV loading dose of 15mg\kg can be given, which takes a few hours to reach therapeutic levels. Plasma levels should be checked if fits are difficult to control.

Carbamazepine (Tegretol) 100mg BD up to 400mg TID, is used to control focal seizures.

Valproate (Epilim) 200-400mg QID is effective for both generalized and focal seizures and has few side-effects. It can be used instead of or with the above drugs.

Midazolam (Hypnovel) is a water soluble benzodiazepine, that can be used in subcutaneous infusions to prevent the recurrence of fits, for patients unable to swallow oral anti-convulsants. It can be mixed with a variety or drugs in an infusion, including diamorphine, cyclizine, haloperidol and hyoscine. The usual dose range is 30-60mg over 24 hours. (It has a half-life of only 3 hours after a single dose). It is also useful to reduce muscle stiffness or multifocal myoclonic twitching in the terminal phase.

Phenobarbitone 100mg BD by IM injection will control seizures in patients unable to swallow anti-convulsants. Water-soluble phenobarbitone can be given as a subcutaneous infusion, 200-600mg a day, but it does not mix with other drugs and has to be given by itself via a second syringe driver.

Explanation is important following a first seizures because the patient and relatives are often frightened. They can be reassured that seizures due to brain tumours rarely affect mental function or prognosis. Teach first-aid to the relatives, including:

- Left lateral position
- Cushion from hard objects
- Do not interfere with the mouth
- Post-ictal drowsiness occurs

SEXUAL PROBLEMS

Physical intimacy continues to be an important need for many cancer patients. Couples usually welcome the opportunity to discuss the effects of the illness on their relationship and their physical intimacy. Patients with cancer continue to need physical contact and sometimes want to continue a sexual relationship.

Useful questions to approach the subject include:

- How has this illness affected your relationship?
- Are you still able to kiss and cuddle?

Communication is often the main problem. Physical illness changes relationships. The effect of illness is very often to reduce communication about feelings (because of tiredness, changed routines, worries about symptoms, medical appointments, medication, increased family pressures).

Assumptions get made about each other's needs and feelings, and these assumptions are often wrong. A short discussion about feelings will often be able to heal misunderstandings ("I thought that he'd gone off me", "We thought it might be dangerous").

SKIN PROBLEMS

Common skin changes in advanced cancer are greyish discolouration of the skin, purpura (thrombocytopenia) and bruising due to steroids.

Rarer skin changes include diffuse pigmentation from ectopic ACTH, vasculitis (tiny purplish lumps on buttocks\legs), urticaria, erythema multiforme (target lesions of concentric rings of erythema), erythema annulare centrifugum (slowly enlarging patches of erythema with a scaly edge) and blistering of the skin (pemphigus\pemphigoid).

Blistering of the skin (bullous lesions) may be due to :

- Staphylococcal infection
- Pemphigus
- Toxic Epidermal Necrolysis

Staphylococcal infection with certain rarer bacterial phage types can produce a toxin, which causes blistering (disseminated bullous impetigo). It is seen quite commonly in children (the scalded skin syndrome) but is very rare in adults. It occurs occasionally in immuno-suppression or advanced cancer.

New lesions appear each day, and since the blisters are fragile and easily rupture they usually appear as superficial erosions (1-5 cm), wherever there has been skin friction. Rubbing the skin may produce a blister (Nikolsky sign). Avoid steroids, take swabs and treat with oral flucloxacillin 500mg QID, and topical mupirocin (Bactroban) ointment, 3 times a day, which is broad spectrum and active against resistant organisms.

Pemphigus (usually with oral lesions) is suspected if the lesions persist despite antibiotics. Consider skin biopsy to diagnose the cause.

Toxic epidermal necrolysis (which is usually a drug reaction and often preceded by target skin lesions of eythema multiforme) can cause a similar blistering eruption. Skin biopsy is needed for diagnosis.

Paraneoplastic dermatoses (rare skin conditions strongly associated with an underlying carcinoma) include:

- Acanthosis nigricans
- Erythema gyratum repens
- Dermatomyositis
- Migratory thrombophlebitis
- Acquired hypertrichosis lanuginosa
- Pachydermo-periostosis

Acanthosis nigricans is a dark velvety rash in the axilla (neck, groin or peri-umbilicus) consisting of small brown or black pigmented warts. A benign form occurs in obesity. 50% have an underlying carcinoma (often gastric) and it signals a short prognosis. Tumour peptides may stimulate growth receptors in the skin.

Erythema gyratum repens is a very rare and dramatic rash, with lines of redness in a woodgrain pattern over most of the body.

Dermatomyositis causes a typical rash on light-exposed areas of skin with muscle tenderness and proximal weakness of the arms. There is a typical rash on the eyelids, arteritic lesions around the nail-beds, and purplish papules over the finger joints. It responds to high dose steroids. At least 20% have an underlying carcinoma (bronchus, breast, stomach, ovary). In males over 50, 60% have carcinoma of the bronchus.

Migratory thrombophlebitis cause intense inflammation of a segment of a vein, subsiding over 2-3 weeks, tending to recur further along the vein. It may be due to disordered fibrinolysis. It is strongly associated with cancers of the pancreas and lung.

Acquired hypertrichosis lanuginosa ("malignant down") is sometimes seen in advanced cancer. It is excessive growth of fine silky hair (resembing the lanugo of babies) over the face and later the rest of the body. The hair growth starts suddenly and grows rapidly. It involves areas which are normally hairless (eyelids, nose). It is distressing and best managed with hair-removing cream (such as Immac).

Pachydermo-periostosis is clubbing (subperiosteal new bone formation) and skin thickening (hands, lips, ears and tongue – which can resemble acromegaly). It can be familial or acquired in men, almost always with lung cancer.

References:
Proby CM, Mortimer PS, Badger C. Non-metastatic manifestations of malignancy: cutaneous. Palliative Medicine 1989; 3: 167-180.
Cox NH, Regnard C. Disseminated bullous impetigo in adult patients with advanced cancer. Palliative Medicine 1991; 5: 66-69.

SMELLS

Smell is embarassing, demoralizing and socially isolating. Anaerobic organisms (especially Bacteroides) were noted to be associated with smell in 1938 in peritonitis. They flourish in necrotic tissue and produce volatile fatty acids, which cause the smell. They are absorbed by charcoal. The de-odorizing effect of metronidazole was reported in 1980.

Treatment options:

- Wound debridement
- Metronidazole orally
- Metronidazole gel
- Air filtration
- Charcoal dressings

Wound debridement to cut off necrotic tissue reduces smell and promotes healing. Small areas can be removed painlessly with scissors.

Oral metronidazole (Flagyl) 200-400mg, TID, reduces the smell of anaerobic infections, usually within 2-3 days. It is useful for smelly cutaneous malignancy (fungation), lung abscess causing foul halitosis, or a necrotic rectal tumour causing a smelly discharge. Continuous treatment (at 200mg 8 hourly) is necessary, as the organisms re-grow. It may cause nausea and can cause severe headaches with alcohol. Longterm use may (rarely) cause a neuropathy.

Chloramphenicol 500mg 6 hourly, will also reduce smell due to anaerobes, and has a place for patients who cannot tolerate metronidazole. It has very few side-effects compared to other broad-spectrum antibiotics active against anaerobes, such as erythromycin and clindamycin.

Metronidazole 0.8% gel (Metrotop) applied daily to fungating skin tumours is soothing and controls smell very effectively in 90% of patients. In a series of 68 patients with a foul-smelling tumour, 34 (50%) reported complete control of odour using the gel, 31 (46%) reported reduced smell and in 3 there was no effect (Newman *et al*, 1989). Improvement usually began within 2 days, but sometimes took a month. 3 found it completely ineffective. Skin irritation occured in 1. It is 30× more expensive that oral metronidazole, and should be reserved for failure to oral metronidazole.

Charcoal dressings help absorb smell, and can be placed on top of other dressings, usually held in place with elastic netting.

Electric air filtration is essential for severe odour problems. A good filter will effectively remove smell from the room. The Bionaire F100 is recommended (available from Clean Air Systems Tel. 0788 823084).

Deodorant sprays are best avoided, as they mix with the smell rather than removing it.

Reference:
Newman V, Allwood M. Oakes RA. The use of metronidazole gel to control the smell of malodorous lesions. Palliative Medicine 1989; 3: 303-305.

SPINAL CORD COMPRESSION

Spinal cord compression occurs in 3-5% of patients with cancer and the frequency is higher in some tumours (15% in myeloma, 10% in prostate cancer). It is a medical emergency. Neurological symptoms can develop rapidly, over a period of hours, and delay in treatment can cause irreversible paralysis. Emergency treatment involves giving 30mg dexamethasone IV immediately and planning same-day radiotherapy.

It is very important to have a high index of suspicion, because once weakness of the legs has occured it is usually too late to restore walking. Most patients have increasing back pain for weeks or months before neurological symptoms occur, and plain Xrays of the spine will demonstrate the presence or absence of extradural tumour in 80% of cases. It is not a fatal complication, and 30% of patients will live 1 year after cord compression, so prevention of paralysis is very important. Patients should be warned about reporting back pain or "tired legs" or "funny feelings" in the legs. Severe back pain that is worse on coughing or lying down is very suspicious. Once signs develop it may be too late to recover function. RT should be considered as a preventative measure whenever thoracic metastases are detected.

The tumours that causes cord compression are most commonly cancers of the lung, breast and prostate, and myeloma. Less commonly it occurs in lymphoma, sarcoma, and cancers of the kidney, thyroid, stomach and colon. Prognosis is better in lymphoma and myeloma.

The mechanism of cord compression in 85% is extradural (epidural) compression, due to direct extension from the vertebral body into the anterior epidural space. Direct spread of a paraspinal tumour mass through the intervertebral foramen is associated with lymphoma and testicular tumours, and this will not be detectable on Xrays but will be on CT scan.

The site of compression is usually thoracic (70%), but can be lumbar (20%) or cervical (10%), and can be multiple. Cervical compression causes quadraparesis and requires surgical fixation. Lumbar compression affects the conus medullaris (which lies between T9-L1) which supplies the lumbar and sacral nerves. Below L1 the cord ends and compression affects the nerve roots (*see Cauda equina compression, below*).

Symptoms of cord compression are back pain and weak legs. 90% will have thoracic back pain sometimes with root pains radiating around both sides of chest and worse on coughing. The weakness may present as difficulty climbing stairs or as stiffness at first. The sensory changes may simply be described as "funny feelings". Urinary hesitancy and peri-anal numbness are a late features. Signs include:

- Thoracic bony tenderness
- Increased leg tone and reflexes.
- Upgoing plantar reflexes
- A sensory level (nipple=T4, umbilicus = T10)
- Urinary retention

Cauda equina compression cause a different clinical picture. The cauda equina ("Horse's tail") is a leash of nerve roots that extend from the end of the spinal cord (L1 verteba) to the intervertebral foramina, where they leave the spinal canal. Compression of these nerve roots causes a similar picture to infiltration of the lumbo-sacral plexus by pelvic tumours:

- Weak legs (flaccid weakness)
- Sciatic pain (often bilateral)
- Urinary hesitancy or retention
- Peri-anal numbness

The diagnosis is difficult to prove (even myelogram may appear normal). Treatment to relieve the compression is with radiotherapy or steroids. Radiotherapy is often disappointing, possibly because of poor localization of the area of compression.

Investigations of spinal cord compression should not delay emergency treatment: X-rays may show eroded pedicles or a collapsed vertebra, CT scan may show a soft tissue epidural mass, but only looks at one level. MRI scan is the investigation of choice prior to surgery, and shows the whole length of the cord, and will show if there are multiple areas of compression, but the patient has to lie still for 30 minutes for the scan. Myelogram may be indicated pre-operatively to show the extent of the block.

Radiotherapy within 48 hours can sometimes restore function, partially or completely. Radiotherapy alone gives as good results as radiotherapy plus laminectomy. RT is most suitable for slowly developing lesions, which respond best. Radiotherapy cannot restore stability to a totally collapsed vertebra, but can reduce bone pain. It is most effective for extradural deposits due to myeloma, leukaemia or lymphoma. A commonly used regime is 3000 cGy in 10 fractions. The level of thoracic pain and sensory level indicate the level for emergency radiotherapy.

The results of RT: 70% of patients who can walk at presentation retain the ability to walk, but only 5% of those who are already paraplegic. Unfortunately most patients present late. Rescue of sphincter function occurs in about 60% of those treated early, and may still be a worthwhile goal, even if legs are already weak. Chemotherapy is of very little benefit.

The dilemma in advanced disease is often whether to refer for radiotherapy at all, since the results of treatment are often disappointing, and several trips to a radiotherapy department may not be in the patient's best interests when life is short and precious. Discussing options and priorities with the patient and family makes the correct decision clearer. Single large fraction treatments are possible but not necessarily optimal.

Surgical decompression is usually only considered if:

- Biopsy is needed (diagnosis uncertain)
- Radiotherapy is not effective
- Tumour is radio-resistant (melanoma, renal)
- Spine unstable (collapse)
- Major structural compression
- Cervical cord lesion

Posterior decompression laminectomy has been the standard approach for many years, but has disappointing results, because most tumours lie anterior to the cord (spreading from the vertebral body). A selective surgical approach is needed.

Vertebral body resection and stabilization of the spine with rods and wiring, gives better results than RT alone or RT combined with posterior laminectomy. In one prospective study of 61 patients following anterior verebral body resection and reconstruction, 80% achieved post-operative ambulation (Seigal 1985). In the thoracic region this involves a standard postero-lateral thoracotomy, but the technique requires considerable expertise and causes significant blood loss.

References:
Kramer JA. Spinal cord compression in malignancy. Palliative Medicine 1992; 6: 202-211.
Seigal T, Seigal T. Current considerations in the management of neoplastic spinal cord compression. Spine 1989; 14(2). 223 8.

SPINAL DRUGS

Opioid receptors in the spinal cord and brain were discovered in 1973. Direct opioid analgesia at spinal receptors was first described experimentally in 1976, and in 1979 intrathecal morphine was shown to produce effective analgesia in man. Selective spinal analgesia, giving morphine directly onto spinal receptors, has the advantage that much lower doses are needed, causing fewer side- effects, and morphine acts on the pain pathway, not peripheral nerves, and does not cause the motor and sensory blockade that occurs when local anaesthetic is given spinally. The spinal route may be epidural or spinal (intrathecal).

Epidural morphine is the delivery of morphine into the epidural space. The main indication is severe pain that cannot be managed with oral or systemic morphine because of unacceptable drowsiness. It is especially useful for severe sciatic pain not controlled by other measures. The epidural catheter is usually inserted at the level of L1. The level is not critical, because the analgesic effect depends on morphine diffusing into the CSF from the epidural space. The free end of the catheter is tunnelled under the skin, to ensure that any skin infection is trivial and does not track down to the epidural space. A long IV catheter can be used to form the tunnel for the epidural catheter to be passed through. Morphine is given through a filter, attached to the free end of the catheter.

The starting dose of morphine is 25% of the 4 hourly oral dose as a bolus injection, or one tenth of the 24 hour subcutaneous dose as a continuous infusion by pump. The dose range for ongoing therapy is usually 5-50mg per 24 hours. The duration of action of a bolus injection is usually about 12 hours, but varies from 4-24 hours. One unanswered question is how much of the analgesic effect is due to the absorbtion of morphine that occurs into the circulation via the epidural veins, but analgesia lasting longer than 2-3 hours after a bolus must be mainly acting directly on spinal receptors. One problem with bolus injections is that they can be very painful in some patients, possibly due to the catheter tip being near a nerve root, and this can be reduced be giving 1ml 2% lignocaine before the injection.

The main disadvantage of an epidural is that the patient has to have a permanent indwelling catheter in the back, which may be connected to a delivery system, usually a Graseby pump. Side effects are unusual, because of the lower doses, but may include nausea, itch (10%), urinary hesitancy and drowsiness (at higher doses). There is some evidence that the addition of dilute local anaesthetic may increase the analgesic effect of spinal morphine, and adding dilute solutions of bupivacaine, such as 0.125% or 0.0625% (usually 20ml 12 hourly) to the morphine may reduce pain sensation without affecting the larger motor fibres, so that leg strength is not lost.

Reference:
Ottesen S, Minton M, Twycross RG, The use of epidural morphine at a palliative care centre, Palliative Medicine 1990; 4: 117-122

Spinal (intrathecal) morphine can have a place in the longterm control of severe pain not controlled by other methods. A test dose of 0.2mg morphine in 2ml saline, is given at L1, and the patient is then kept in a semi-sitting position for 4 hours. If good pain control is achieved for at least 12 hours, then a permanent intrathecal catheter and subcutaneous system can be implanted. Intrathecal doses are about a tenth of epidural doses. Most patients require between 1-5mg morphine every 12-24 hours to maintain the analgesic effect.

The main risk of the spinal route is infection and therefore implantable systems have been developed. Some have a subcutaneous portal (e.g. Port-A-Cath) which require regular injections every 12-24 hours through the skin. Other systems can provide a continuous infusion either from a reservoir, usually implanted in the gluteal region (which can function for several weeks) or an implantable pump, re-filled every few weeks, but these systems are very expensive. The system can remain effective for many months, the main complications being CSF infection and rarely leakage. Respiratory depression is not a problem if small doses are used and the dose is titrated to the patient's pain.

Intraventricular catheters, via a burr hole, have been sucessfully used to control intractable head and neck or facial (trigeminal) pain, but are only indicated in the very rare situation of the spinal CSF circulation being blocked by an epidural metastasis, because CSF circulation rapidly distributes spinal morphine throughout the CSF and reaches the brain within 6 hours.

References:
Gonzalez-Navarro A, et al. Cancer pain and intrathecal morphine, Palliative Medicine, 1989; 3: 287-292.

Intrathecal (spinal) local anaesthetic is a last resort for a patient with uncontrolled pelvic or leg pain. The patient loses power and sensation in the legs and needs to be catheterized. It has a place if a patient is already paraplegic or bedbound and catheterized. Following the procedure, as the pain disappears, the dose of morphine needs to be reduced or stopped, therefore the patient should be on 4 hourly morphine rather than MST at the time the procedure is performed. In one case a 65 year old woman with a sacral chordoma had good pain relief for 9 weeks, and the dose of lignocaine remained at 4mg per hour without tolerance developing. Test injections of fentanyl confirmed that the pain was not opioid responsive. Pressure sores on the heels healed, partly due to better nursing care made possible by the pain relief and probably partly due to the improved circulation due to sympathetic blockade.

Reference:
Hardy PAJ Wells JCD, Continuous intrathecal lignocaine infusion analgesia: a case report of a nine-week "spinal", Palliative Medicine 1989; 3: 23-25

Epidural clonidine has sucessfully controlled pain in patients with spinal cord injury when epidural morphine was not effective. In some cases pain control was maintained with oral clonidine (Glyn et al, Lancet 1986; ii: 1249-50).

Further reading:
Cherry DA, Gourlay GK The spinal administration of opioids in the treatment of acute and chronic pain: bolus doses, continuous infusions, intraventricular administration and implanted drug delivery systems, Palliative Medicine 1987; 1: 89-106.

SPIRITUAL PAIN

What is spiritual pain? Dame Cicely Saunders describes spiritual pain like this: "The realization that life is likely to end soon may well stimulate a desire to put first things first and to reach out to what is seen as true and valuable – and to give rise to feelings of being unable or unworthy to do so. There may be bitter anger at the unfairness of what is happening, and at much of what has gone before, and above all a desolating feeling of meaninglessness. Here lies, I believe, the essence of spiritual pain." (Hospital Chaplain, March 1988).

Spiritual or religious? Everyone has a spiritual part to them, but not everyone is religious. Religion provides a framework of beliefs and rituals to express spiritual concerns. Spiritual support is grounded in the ordinary. For example pleasant surroundings, with sunlight, flowers, trees, clean comfortable furniture and pleasant smells can all uplift the spirit, and are part of routine spiritual support.

The experience of illness can make previous attitudes and assumptions about life (past, present and future) seem suddenly redundant. But a crisis is not an entirely negative experience. It feels dangerous but it is also an opportunity for change. Lily Pincus in her book "Death and the Family" goes so far as to say "A crisis is not an abstract imposition from without, but a high point in the life of the person concerned ... a dynamic interaction between a person and an extreme event". Many patients tell how their appreciation of life has been deepened because of their illness. A patient is not (usually) responsible for their illness but is ultimately responsible for their reaction to being ill and facing death.

Recognizing spiritual pain is difficult. We tend to ignore or play down painful comments like "I seem to be wasting away" or "I've led a good life" or "I feel a burden" because they threaten to lead on to a discussion which will be distressing to us, at a deep level, as well as the patient. And yet for most people the spiritual questions are the most important ones. The questions may be about illness:

- Why me?
- Why now?
- Why this illness?

or questions about life:

- Guilt (past)
- Isolation (present)
- Hopelessness or Fear (future)

Providing spiritual support cannot be entirely separated from the routine care and support given to patients. Spiritual distress has a habit of emerging in intimate and relaxing moments – such as provided by a bed-bath or a hair-do or a massage. What else can we do to help? It is tempting to image that since we have a certain expertise, we also possess the means to take away spiritual distress as well. But we are unlikely to be experts in suffering, and can never be experts in another person's suffering. The patient is going ahead of us on a shared journey. All we can do is listen and try to offer empathy and companionship. Trying to rescue patients from their distress would be to devalue their experience. But true empathy, an attempt to understand another person's suffering, can be very healing. One of the most helpful comments about offering spiritual support is this: "It is definitely more important to clarify the depth of the questions than to give their right answers" (Rivera-Reyes). Listening can often bring a partial resolution of anguish over time (*see Counselling*)

Companionship is at the heart of real spiritual support ("It is not theology they want, its you") and yet it is difficult to define the quality that is needed. To quote Jean Vanier: "In some mysterious way, the quality of my presence, my look, brings to you life – or death". The most hoped for companion for the sick or dying patient may be a family member, but a comparative stranger can also bring support and encouragement. A real companion will quietly and genuinely try to understand.

The unconcious part of the mind, particularly obvious in remembered dreams, can make available to our conscious mind valuable information about ourselves. Ann Faraday, in her book Dream Power says "... when rational thought relaxes control during sleep, the day's background chatter comes to the fore ... this chatter is the source of much creative activity, as associations and ideas spread through the mind and link with new trains of thought and feeling. In this way new and unexpected connections are made, giving fresh meanings to old ideas. Metaphors, slang, puns, overlapping meanings and figures of speech are the language used by the chattering mind to create new forms of mental life, of which the dream is only one".

3 Methods of providing spiritual support will be described which can encourage the integration of the unconcious and the conscious parts of the mind:

- Imagework
- Art Therapy
- Reminiscence

Imagework has similarities to some forms of hypnotherapy, and is a method of using unconscious images to help the patient to integrate their unconscious understanding and become more comfortable with their experiences. After inducing a state of deep relaxation, the patient is encouraged to form visual images of various aspects of their physical or emotional distress, e.g. "I want you to imagine a picture that describes your experience at the moment" and then, perhaps, "If the image could speak, what would it say?" or "If you could change places with the image, what would you see?" This method of using dialogue can enable the patient to "see things differently". This type of therapy needs to be practised by an experienced therapist who is familiar with (and has experienced) this technique and is able to cope with the powerful emotions that may be released. This method can sucessfully allow a patient to reach some peace of mind when other methods fail. (Reference: Kearney M. Imagework in a case of intractable pain. Palliative Medicine 1992; 6: 152-157.)

Art therapy can be a powerful way of enabling a search for meaning to occur. Visual images can communicate what words cannot, and they can bring relief, understanding and even sometimes surprise. They allow a reaching into the unconscious, where images can function as a means of integration. Art therapy can contribute to the patient's well-being and answers the fundamental human need to be creative. An art therapist can encourage a reluctant patient to "experiment with and experience and enjoy colours" to help overcome any embarrassment about somehow failing to produce something which is acceptable "art". The art therapist is also trained to stay alongside the emotional turmoil that may be released at times. "Non-artistic" people may find this method particularly helpful. On a personal note, some years ago I painted the only pictures I have ever painted as an adult, over a period of 4 days, either side of a conversion experience. I felt suddenly compelled to paint, not knowing beforehand what images I would produce, and the pictures communicated something important and new to me. Other types of art therapy that may be suitable for particular individuals may include using sculpture or poetry. (Reference: Connell C. Art Therapy as part of a palliative care programme. Palliative Medicine 1992; 6: 18-25).

Reminiscence is a natural and enjoyable pastime, but can also be especially helpful at the end of life. The patient is encouraged to talk about their early family life, parent, siblings, upbringing, schooling, friends, hobbies, work and achievements. This simple (but time-consuming) technique has several benefits. It is a way of remembering life experiences, integrating present experiences into the context of a whole life. The North American indian chief Crazy Horse said "Today is a good day to die, for all the things of my life are present". Encouraging reminiscence also helps a patient to feel known as themselves and emphasizes a person's uniqueness. In his book "Man's Search for Meaning" Victor Frankl emphasises the spiritual strength and sense of meaning that can be derived from memories of past loves and past achievements. The formal encouraging of memories can be called "Reminiscence Therapy". One method is to specifically employ a person with interviewing and listening skills, who can tape record the life-story and can later transcribe some of the conversations. These can be given to the patient, or the family, and extracts can also be collected into an archive and published as booklets – adding to the creativity of the process.

Religious rituals are extremely important to some patients as they near the time of their death. Religious beliefs and rituals are intended to provide a positive way of responding to and making sense of questions about the meaning of life. Rituals do not have to be formal, and sacraments can be given at the bedside in a way that is personalized and fitting to the patient's needs. For some people religious beliefs, sacraments and symbols provide important and sustaining spiritual support, but they cannot entirely replace the need for human contact and empathy. The Christian faith can offer particular comfort to the dying. Images of God are so often punitive for many people, and yet the heart of the Christian message is that Christ was also trapped in human suffering and yet through the resurrection also offers us hope for meaning beyond death.

Recommended further reading:
Mud and Stars. The impact of Hospice Experience on the Church's Ministry of Healing. Report of a Working Party. 1991 Sobell Publications. (246 pages).
Lichter I, Mooney J, Boyd M. Biography as Therapy. Palliative Medicine 1993; 7: 133–137

STEROIDS

Steroid hormones are synthesized by the adrenal glands. There are 3 types:

- Glucocorticoids   –   cortisol (hydrocortisone)
- Mineralocorticoids   –   aldosterone
- Sex hormones   –   androgens, oestrogens, progestagens

Glucocorticoids convert proteins to glucose (and steroids therefore pre-dispose to diabetes) and are powerfully anti-inflammatory by inhibiting phospholipase and decreasing prostaglandin synthesis. Mineralocorticoids cause sodium retention.

Steroids and cancer. In 1943 steroids were reported to cause lymphoid atrophy in mice and shortly after were shown to cause regression of lymphoid tumours. Steroids improve the response rate to chemotherapy in myeloma and breast cancer, but have not been found to have a specific role in the treatment of other solid cancers.

Steroids in palliative medicine are widely used to control symptoms. In a series of 373 hospice patients, 50% received steroids for a variety of reasons and 40% derived some benefit from them. 5% had to stop them due to side-effects. (Hanks *et al* 1983). In a randomized double-blind cross-over trial in 40 patients with advanced cancer, steroids significantly reduced pain, depression and anorexia, but the effect wore off in 34% of patients within 4-5 weeks (Bruera 1985). Steroids reduce peri-tumour oedema and relieve compression. The mechanism for many of their actions (e.g. appetite stimulant, reducing cerebral oedema, anti-emetic, feeling of well-being) are not understood. Give steroids early in the day to prevent insomnia. The main clinical uses are given in the table.

Clinical uses of steroids are:

CLINICAL PROBLEM	USUAL DAILY DOSE
Anorexia	4mg
SVC compression Lymphangitis Malignant dysphagia Pyloric obstruction Nerve pain Intractable nausea	8mg
Cord compression Brain metastases	16mg

Anorexia is improved significantly more by steroids (80%) than by placebo (50%), although the high placebo response emphasizes the importance of psychological factors (Willox *et al*. Prednisolone as an appetite stimulant in patients in patients with cancer. Br Med J 1984; 288:27).

Which steroid?

EQUIVALENT ANTI-INFLAMMATORY DOSES:	
Cortisone acetate	30mg
Hydrocortisone	30mg
Prednisonlone	7mg
Triamcinolone	5mg
Betamethasone	1mg
Dexamethasone	1mg

Cortisone is inactive until converted to hydrocortisone (cortisol) in the liver. Hydrocortisone is unsuitable for longterm therapy because of its sodium retaining properties. Prednisolone is as effective as dexamethasone. Dexamethasone has negligible mineralocorticoid activity. There are no controlled studies to compare the effectiveness of steroids in controlling symptoms, but a prospective analysis of 250 hospice patients showed no difference in efficacy or side-effects, except that dexamethasone was more likely to cause restlessness.

Dexamethasone is the most commonly used steroid in symptom control because of its potency. 2mg of dexamethasone is equivalent to 15mg of prednisolone. Dexamethasone is methyl-fluoro-prednisolone and is metabolized more slowly than other steroids, with a plasma half-life of 3-6 hours. It has negligible mineralocorticoid activity.

N.B. Phenytoin and carbamezepine reduce the effectiveness of dexamethasone by 50% (because hepatic enzyme induction increases metabolism).

The oral route is as effective as the IV or SC route. A steady plasma level is achieved after 24 hours. IV steroids are only indicated in emergencies (SVC or cord compression). Subcutaneous dexamethasone can be mixed with a variety of other drugs (*see Subcutaneous Infusions*).

A trial of high dose steroids is often indicated in symptom control. Steroids are given for 7-10 days. If the symptom improves, the high dose is continued but may need to be reduced after a time to avoid side-effects (especially facial swelling), in which case it should be reduced gradually (e.g. 2mg every 1 or 2 weeks), to prevent the symptom recurring. Explain the purpose and possible side-effects of steroids to the patient and family, and that a marked improvement in symtoms does not mean tumour regression.

Side-effects of steroids become more likely the longer treatment continues, but only 5% of patients have to stop steroids because of severe side-effects.

- Oral thrush (40%)
- Facial disfigurement (30%)
- Oedema (20%)
- Mental agitation (8%)
- Dyspepsia (5%)
- Diabetes (5%)
- Weight gain (4%)
- Insomnia (3%)

Less common side-effects of steroids:

- Hyperphagia (distressing appetite)
- Myopathy
- Abdominal distension
- Worsening of cataracts
- Re-activation of tuberculosis
- Acne
- Striae
- Myoclonic jerks
- Osteoporosis

Oral thrush is common and prophylactic anti-fungal treatment should be started with steroids. Facial disfigurement (swelling, rapid hair growth) is the most distressing problem and is sometimes severe. Diabetes can be treated with oral hypoglycaemics. Known diabetics will need an increase in insulin dosage. Myopathy affects the proximal leg muscles (difficulty standing up from a chair or climbing stair). Abdominal distension is partly due to re-distribution of fat, partly to wasting and weakness of abdominal muscles and possibly also colonic distension. Tuberculosis may be re-activated, but in a cancer patient with recent TB steroids can usually be safely given if covered by treatment with Rifinah 300 (rifampicin 300mg plus isoniazid 150mg).

Peptic ulceration (gastric or duodenal) is often feared, but a large case control study has shown that it occurs with no higher frequency in patients on steroids than other cancer patients, unless the patient is also taking an NSAID, when the risk is doubled. Patients on both steroids and NSAIDs should therefore also take an acid inhibitor such as ranitidine or a gastro-protective agent such as misoprostol (see Dyspepsia). (Piper J et al. 1991).

Steroid psychosis is rare. About 20% on high dose steroids experience insomnia, restlessness, agitation or elation. These usually start within 1-2 days of starting steroids, and can occur at low doses, such as dexamethasone 2mg daily (prednisolone 15mg). Psychotic features such as mania, euphoria, pressure of speech, grandiose ideas or paranoia can all occur rarely, but there are usually warning signs of restlessness and agitation. They occur after 2-3 weeks and are unusual with doses below 6mg dexamthasone. Management involves reducing the dose of steroids and starting haloperidol 5mg 12 hourly (or chlorpromazine 100-150mg 6 hourly if there is a lot of agitation) and then gradually reducing the sedation over a period of days as the patient responds. One study (Hanks 1983) suggested that dexamethasone is more likely that prednisolone to cause psychological disturbances. Tricyclics are known to worsen steroid-induced syndromes. (Reference: Bell G et al. Cerebral metastases and dexamethasone: psychiatric aspects; Palliative Medicine 1987; 1: 132-135).

Stopping steroids can be done rapidly if they have been given for less than 1 week, because there is no risk of adrenal suppression. If the patient has been on high dose steroids longer than 1 week the dose must be reduced very gradually (down to 0.5mg prednisolone alternate days) before stopping, to avoid an adrenal crisis and hypotension.

Replacement steroids are needed by patients with pituitary or adrenal failure or adrenal suppression by aminoglutethamide. Hydrocortisone 20-40mg daily has both glucocorticoid and mineralocorticoid activity and is adequate unless there is primary adrenal failure when fludrocortisone 50-200 micrograms daily is also needed. Dexamethasone 1mg daily provides adequate glucocorticoid replacement but has little mineral-ocorticoid activity. Therefore if a patient on replacement steroids is started on dexamethasone they should stay on their normal replacement steroids as well, otherwise sodium loss and hypotension can occur.

The treatment of cerebral oedema with steroids is of most benefit for metastatic tumours and high grade astrocytomas, and is of less use for slow-growing, infiltrating tumours. It is reasonable to start with 16mg dexamethasone daily. (see Brain metastases for a detailed discussion of the use of steroids in cerebral oedema).

Rectal steroids are useful to control diarrhoea due to rectal tumours or radiation proctitis. Preparations include:

- Predsol suppository (5mg prednisolone)
- Colifoam (125mg hydrocortisone) – 5ml
- Predfoam (20mg prednisolone) – 20ml
- Predsol enema (20mg prednisolone) – 100ml

The suppository acts in the rectum, the foams pass up to the descending colon, the enema reaches higher but is difficult to retain. Colifoam is usually the most convenient, being only 5ml, and comes in a 14 dose aerosol with a re-usable rectal applicator. Some patients prefer the predfoam delivery system with disposable rectal nozzles.

Local steroid injections of methlyprednisolone (Depomedrone) given under local anaesthetic can be used to control rib pain or can be given epidurally for vertebral pain (*see Nerve Blocks*).

References:
Twycross R. Corticosteroids in advanced cancer. Br Med J. 24 Oct 1992; Vol 305: 969–970
Hanks GW, Trueman T, Twycross RG, Corticosteroids in advanced cancer – a prospective analysis of current practice. Postgraduate Medical Journal, November 1983, 59, 702-706.
Piper JM, Ray WA, Daughterty JR, Griffin MR. Corticosteroid use and peptic ulcer disease: role of nonsteroidal anti-inflammatory drugs. Ann Intern Med 1991; 114: 735-40.
Bruera E *et al*, Action of oral methylprednisolone in terminal cancer patients: a prospective randomized trial. Cancer Treat Rep 1985; 69: 751-54.

STOMACH CANCER

Stomach cancer causes around 10,500 deaths per year in the UK. It usually presents with a long history of dyspepsia. Diagnosis is by gastroscopy and biopsy. Curative surgery is attempted in 40%, but only 10% are cured, because even superficial-looking lesions may have already spread to the nodes. Radical gastrectomy is followed by gastro-jejunostomy (if a stomach remnant can be left) or oesophago-jejunostomy. Post-operatively the patient requires iron, B12 therapy (and penicillin after splenectomy). A mass, nodes or ascites suggest advanced disease, when survival is measured in months.

Palliative resection (partial gastrectomy and gastro-jejunostomy) may be attempted to reduce the problems or pain or obstruction, but operative mortality is high. Intubation can be offered for obstructive lesions in the fundus. Metastases occur to liver and sometimes lung. Radiotherapy has no place, causing severe nausea and not improving survival.

Chemotherapy may be considered to control symptoms. 5FU (with or without folinic acid) has about a 20% response rate. Other drugs that are known to be effective, used alone or in combination, include doxorubicin, mitomycin and cisplatin, although the toxicity of cisplatin makes it unsuitable for most of these patients. Prolonged chemotherapy infusions may increase the response rate, but at the cost of more side-effects.

Problems in advanced cancer of the stomach include:

- Pain
- Dyspepsia (Ranitidine)
- Pyloric stenosis
- Ascites
- Steatorrhoea

Pain is epigastric and may radiate into the back. A coeliac plexus block should be considered early for pain that is not responding to morphine. Dyspepsia may respond to ranitidine.

Pyloric stenosis causes a high intestinal obstruction and vomiting. 50% will get relief of vomiting with high dose steroids (*see Nausea and Vomiting*).

Steatorrhoea may occur due to invasion of the pancreas by posterior tumours and blockage of the pancreatic duct. It responds to pancreatic supplements (*see Diarrhoea*).

STOMAS

A stoma is a surgically created opening of the bowel or urinary tract on to the body surface.

End stomas are the simplest to create. The bowel is divided and brought to the surface of the skin. They are also called defunctioning stomas. A common example is the sigmoid colostomy after abdomino-perineal excision of the rectum. The end colostomy usually discharges sollid faeces intermittently. The distal end of a divided segment of bowel can be closed and returned to the abdomen as in Hartmann's procedure, or brought to the abdominal surface and sutured to the skin, and it is then termed a mucus fistula.

Loop stomas are usually temporary and are formed when a mobile loop of bowel, usually transverse colon, is brought up to the surface, and a hole is cut in the bowel and sutured to the skin. They are used to decompress the bowel to relieve obstruction, or to protect a segment of bowel with an anastomosis. Generally, the intention is to reverse the colostomy at a later date. In advanced disease a loop colostomy may not be reversed, and these colostomies can be difficult to manage, because they are large and irregular and prone to leakage. Some faeces may still pass PR.

An end ileostomy, usually situated in the right iliac fossa, is most commonly performed following total excision of the colon for ulcerative colitis. Ileostomy contents are semi-liquid and will digest and excoriate unprotected skin. For this reason the ileostomy should be constructed with a short spout, so that it protrudes into a stoma bag.

An Ileal conduit is most commonly constructed after removal of the bladder. A segment of ileum, still attached to its blood supply, is isolated to act as a reservoir, and brought out as a stoma. The ureters are implanted into it. A drainable appliance allows emptying without removing the bag.

N.B. Suppositories are not retained by a stoma, but a diazepam enema (Stesolid) is usually effective via a stoma.

The stoma appliance that is well fitted is the key to successful management. A one piece system simply consists of a bag which is adhesive. A two-piece system is easier initially, when an adhesive base plate can be cut precisely by a nurse to fit the stoma, and the patient only needs to change the bag, which clips onto the base plate with a ring of plastic. A specialist stoma nurse should advise on the most suitable appliance. The patient needs manual dexterity to change the bag.

Irrigation can be used to manage colostomies, instead of wearing a bag, and is widely practised in the USA. 1.5 litres of warm water is instilled slowly and then runs out with the faecal residue via a disposable system into the toilet. A gauze dressing is then worn over the stoma. Colostomy plugs can sometimes be used, to avoid the use of a bag for about 8 hours, allowing flatus to escape through a filter (Lancet 1986; ii: 1062-3).

Peri-stomal inflammation may be due to a contact <u>allergy to the appliance</u> or <u>effluent dermatitis</u> due to an ill-fitting appliance. Secondary skin infection can occur. Change the appliance, use stomahesive paste to protect the skin and karaya gum to fill in irregularities in the skin.

Surgical problems include:

- Prolapse
- Para-stomal hernia
- Bleeding
- Obstruction

<u>Prolapse</u> of the mucosa can occur, usually with loop colostomies. It looks alarming and unsightly, but is rarely dangerous. It should be reduced by hand as a first aid measure. Surgery is required to close or re-fashion the stoma. Only if the mucosa becomes purple or black is there a risk of intestinal ischaemia and necrosis, and prompt surgery is then required.

<u>Parastomal hernia</u> (a bulge at one side of the stoma) may require repair and re-siting of the stoma if it is causing difficulty fitting the appliance or intermittent obstruction.

<u>Bleeding</u> is usually trivial due to mucosal irritation, and stops with local pressure applied with gauze. Persistent bleeding suggests a stomal secondary deposit, when local cryosurgery can help.

<u>Obstruction</u> may be due to stenosis, impacted faeces, adhesions or malignant involvement.

STRIDOR

Stridor means noisy inspiration due to upper airways obstruction. The cause may be a tumour of the pharynx or larynx or mediastinal lymphadenopathy. The clinical picture includes:

- Difficulty breathing
- Intercostal rescession
- Cyanosis (hypoxia)
- Tachycardia
- Confusion
- Panic

Management options for stridor include:

- Steroids
- Radiotherapy
- Laser
- Stent (for extrinsic compression)
- Tracheostomy

A tracheostomy is stoma into the trachea. After an emergency tracheostomy for stridor, the larynx is left in place and the patient is usually still able to speak by covering the hole (or inserting a speaking tube with a valve) to block exhaled air and re-direct it through the larynx. For the first 2-3 weeks after a tracheostomy there is a risk that the pre-tracheal tissues will close over the stoma if the tube is removed or falls out. The tube is therefore taped in and a pair of tracheal dilators are kept near at hand. The outer tube, which is normally changed every week, needs to be changed quickly at this early stage; after a few weeks the track remains open even when the tube is removed. The inner tube needs removing 2-3 times a day for cleaning, depending on the amount of secretions. Suction is usually only needed for the first few weeks until the patient learns how to cough up secretions, or if the patient has a chest infection, when a portable suction machine may be needed, plus a supply of sterile suction catheters. Skin care simply involves the use of vaseline around the stoma to prevent the skin drying out. Crusts can be softened by breathing humidified air. A piece of foam can be worn over the stoma to prevent sputum exploding out when coughing.

Laryngectomy leaves a wider stoma and no tube is required, except in the post-operative period. The patient has to learn oesophageal speech or uses a vibrator to amplify lip speech.

SUBCUTANEOUS INFUSIONS

A continuous subcutaneous infusion achieves a steady plasma concentration of drugs that is equivalent to an intravenous infusion. It removes the need for regular suppositories or injections.

SC infusions arc indicatcd for:

- Nausea or vomiting
- Intestinal obstruction
- Dysphagia
- Unconsiousness
- Malabsorbtion causing poor pain control

The following drugs arc commonly uscd, and the common starting dose per 24 hours is given:

DRUGS FOR SUBCUTANEOUS INFUSION		
	Starting dose per 24 hours	Ampoule strength
Diamorphine	15mg*	
Haloperidol	5-10mg	5mg\ml
Cyclizine	150mg	50mg\ml
Metoclopramide	40mg	5mg\ml
Methotrimeprazine	75mg	25mg\ml
Hyoscine	1.2mg	0.4mg\ml
Buscopan	60mg	20mg\ml
Midazolam	20mg	5mg\ml
Dexamethasone	4mg	5mg\ml

*__The starting dose of diamorphine__ of 15mg is for a patient who is morphine-naive, i.e. who has not been given morphine before. The 24 hour dose for a patient already pain-controlled on oral morphine would be half the 24 hour oral dose of morphine. For example, a patient who is pain-controlled on MST 60mg BD, would require 60mg of subcutaneous diamorphine per 24 hours. The recommended maximum dose of diamorphine is 250mg\ml, but doses up to 400mg\ml arc possiblc. Diamorphine has been shown to be compatible for 24 hours with cyclizine, haloperidol, metoclopramide, methotrimeprazine, midazolam and hyoscine, but studies have only used moderate doses of 50-150mg\ml of diamorphine.

Other drugs that have been used in SC infusions include octreotide, ondansetron, diclofenac, keterolac, pamidronate and salbutamol. Sodium naproxen has been sucessfully used in a subcutaneous infusion alone or combined with morphine (Palliative Medicine 1989; 3: 207-211). The compatibility of many of these drugs in combination remains unknown. Further research is needed.

The control of nausea and vomiting may require high doses of anti-emetics initially, after which the doses can be gradually reduced over a period of days. It is then often possible to transfer the patient back to oral anti-emetics over a further period of days, starting the oral drugs before stopping the infusion and use high oral doses initially. Methotrimeprazine 100-200mg can be used for very severe nausea or vomiting. Cyclizine 150mg (which acts at cholinergic receptors) and haloperidol 5mg (which acts at dopamine receptors) can be logically combined. Dexamethasone has an anti-emetic effect, and can be safely added to any of the above. Diamorphine and\or Buscopan can also be added to infusions of any of these anti-emetics.

Common situations requiring SC infusion are:

- Nausea or vomiting: diamorphine (if the patient was on oral morphine) with cyclizine or metoclopramide. Dexamethasone may be added (but at higher doses tends to precipitate with cyclizine or haloperidol).
- Intestinal obstruction: diamorphine, cyclizine and buscopan (*see Intestinal obstruction*).
- Terminal phase: diamorphine, methotrimeprazine (Nozinan) and hyoscine (*see Terminal Phase*).

Precipitation or cloudiness of the mixture is an indication to discard the mixture since it indicates partial inactivation of the drugs (and possibly toxic byproducts). Precipitation of drugs may occur at higher doses, (especially diamorphine above 10mg\ml with cyclizine above 10mg\ml). Increase the dilution of the mixture or use two syringe drivers.

Commonly used drugs in SC infusions are:

Cyclizine (100-150mg per 24 hours) is a very useful anti-emetic for gastro-intestinal causes of vomiting or raised ICP. It can precipitate with the hydrochloride in saline, diamorphine, metoclopramide and midazolam.

Metoclopramide (30-100mg per 24 hours) is very effective and has the advantage of causing no drowsiness. It can usefully be combined with cyclizine. It has been safely used in doses as high as 240mg per 24 hours to control chemotherapy-induced vomiting.

Methotrimeprazine (Nozinan, 25-200mg per 24 hours is a powerful anti-emetic for severe nausea, but is very sedating (useful for terminal agitation). Patients with severe nausea will accept some sedation for a few days if explained, and once nausea is controlled the dose can be gradually reduced, and usually the nausea remains controlled.

Haloperidol (3-15mg per 24 hours) is a powerful anti-emetic with little sedation, especially useful if control of restlessness or paranoia is also needed.

Hyoscine hydrobromide (1.2-3.6mg per 24 hours) is useful to dry up secretions or for additional sedation.

Hyoscine butylbromide (Buscopan) 30-80mg per 24 hours, is very useful for colicky pain, and is less sedating than ordinary hyoscine hydrobromide.

Midazolam (Hypnovel) 10-100mg per 24 hours is a water-soluble benzodiazepine, useful to control anxiety, agitation, muscle spasms or as an anti-convulsant, to prevent the recurrence of seizures.

Patient-controlled analgesia (PCA) is a possibility using a subcutaneous infusion and one of the sophisticated (and expensive) pumps available. However, the aim of pain control is to abolish pain in the simplest way possible, so that the patient is able to forget the pain and get back on with his or her life, as far as possible. PCA tends to focus attention on the pain. If a simple and cheap PCA device were available, it may have a place in controlling variable visceral pains, such as pelvic pain that is often much worse on sitting. Most variable pains are due to bone or nerve pain and are only partially morphine-responsive.

The Graseby Syringe Pump MS26 (with the green label) is recommended. It is light (175 grams with battery) and small (16 X 2 X 5cm) and simple to operate. It is designed to give a 24 hour infusion. The rate is measured in mm per 24 hour. (e.g. if the barrel length of medication in the syringe is 45mm, the rate is set for 45, and the entire syringe-full will then be infused over 24 hours). Other equipment that is needed includes small transparent dressing (e.g. Opsite), cotton wool, antiseptic, 10ml or 20ml syringe and prescription from doctor.

Technique of starting an infusion:

1. Discuss site with patient – the butterfly can be sited anywhere, but the anterior chest, abdomen, or thigh are usually the best places. If the patient is restless or confused, place the butterfly on the upper back, where the patient cannot interfere with it.

2. Draw up drugs into syringe, making up the volume if necessary with either sterile water for injection or normal saline. It is better to use water if cyclizine is diluted. Prime the infusion tube (0.75ml) before measuring the barrel length of the medication to be infused. Check there is no clouding of the drugs (crystalization).

3. Measure the length of the infusion in the syringe (different types of syringe have different diameters) – using the ruler on one side of the pump, and set the rate, e.g. 48mm per 24 hours. Then secure the syringe on top of the pump, using the rubber strap. N.B. Never tape the syringe down to the pump – the rubber strap is adequate, and when changing the rate use the small red plastic screwdriver provided, or a paperclip, but never use scissors which often cause expensive damage.

4. Clean the site with antiseptic and insert the butterfly under the skin, and fix down by covering with a small square of Opsite or other transparent dressing, which allows inspection of the site. If the patient is allergic to these dressings use hypoallergenic tape. Secure a loop of cannula with adhesive tape to avoid pull on needle.

5. Start the pump by pressing the start button. The light flashes every 25 seconds. If it is flashing there is enough battery power left to complete that infusion. The 9V PP3 alkaline long-life battery will last for 54 full syringes (don't use rechargeable batteries).

6. The volume infused is usually 20ml per 24 hours, but 2ml per hour (50 ml per day) is absorbed subcutaneously with no swelling at all. In fact, water can be infused subcutaneously into the abdominal wall at a rate of 50ml per hour, with some swelling, but often no discomfort.

7. Warn the patient and relatives that the pump normally beeps from time to time, (indicating 0.23 mm of plunger travel) and that if it blocks or runs out there will be a 10 second warning beep and the pump will stop. The pump is easily portable. A carrying case or belt holster are available, but a "bum-bag" with a zip is safer and easier. Be careful not to immerse the pump in water when washing or bathing. It is generally best to ignore the boost button.

8. Check the site daily for any inflammation or swelling. The site usually needs changing every 2-3 days if the infusion contains anti-emetics, but infusions with diamorphine alone can last several weeks. If the site is not inflamed it can be left alone.

9. Swelling or soreness of the site can be lessened by putting 1-2mg of dexamethasone in the infusion, or if it is severe, 1 ampoule (1500 units) of hyaluronidase (Hyalase) powder can be added to the infusion (provided there is no history of allergy or asthma). Hyalase is an enzyme that lyses connective tissue and increases the permeabilty or the infusion.

Note: A "bum-bag" with a zip is a very useful carrier and easier to use than the holster provided.

Graseby pumps and the infusion sets (60cm or 100cm, with attached butterfly needles) are available from:

> Graseby Medical Ltd
> Colonial Way
> Watford
> Herts, England, WD2 4LG
> Tel 0923 246434 Telex 929263

References:
Oliver DJ. Syringe drivers in palliative care: a review. Palliative Medicine 1988; 2: 21-26.
Johnson I, Patterson S, Drugs used in combination in the syringe driver – a survey of hospice practice. Palliative Medicine 1992; 6: 125-130.

SUPPORT

A crisis means a temporary inability to cope with a new situation. When a new problem arises, new solutions need to be found, and new skills learned. Learning to care for a sick relative is a good example. Several different approaches may need to be tried, before the right solutions are found. Finding new solutions in order to adjust to the new situation involves mental energy ("worry work"), and this process is facilitated by providing additional support for a time.

Supportive behaviour involves:

- Warmth and empathy
- Practical help
- Interpreting new information
- Rehearsing problems
- Toleration of abnormal behaviour (regression)
- Mediation between family members
- Encouraging rest.

SURGERY

Palliative surgery is occasionally indicated, even in far advanced disease:

PROBLEM	PROCEDURE
Dysphagia	Oesophageal tube
Obstruction	Colostomy
Fistula	Colostomy
Ascites	Peritoneovenous shunt
Jaundice	Biliary stent
Fracture	Internal fixation
Skin fungation	Excision, grafting

Good Communication between the surgeon and palliative carers is essential. The patient and family usually need detailed explanation of risks and benefits and the reasons why surgery is being considered at this late stage, and that the surgery is not intended to be curative.

SVC Obstruction

SVC Obstruction (SVCO) is due to compression (or invasion) of the SVC by mediastinal nodes or tumour at the right main bronchus. The SVC drains venous blood from the head and neck and upper thorax (including trachea) to the right atrium .

SVCO is a sub-acute emergency, since without treatment it can progress over a period of several days to a fatal complication.

Tumours that cause SVCO are most commonly lung cancers (mostly small cell) – 75% and lymphomas – 15%. Cancers that cause the other 10% of cases are breast, colon, oesophagus and testis.

Symptoms of SVCO are due to <u>venous hypertension</u> and include dyspnoea (tracheal oedema), headaches (cerebral oedema), visual changes, dizziness (fainting, siezures), swelling of face, neck and arms (tight collar and rings) and a hoarse voice (pressure on recurrent laryngeal nerve). <u>Signs</u> include pink eyes, peri-orbital oedema, dilated neck veins (non-pulsatile) and dilated collateral veins (chest, arms). Late signs may include pleural effusion, pericardial effusion and stridor.

Diagnosis of SVCO is confirmed by a CXR which shows widening of the mediastinum and by CT scan. Further investigations may be needed to provide a tissue diagnosis (for patients who have first presented with SVC obstruction), and may include biopsy of a supraclavicular node, bronchoscopy, mediastinoscopy or even thoracotomy).

Emergency treatment is only needed for advanced SVCO and involves sitting the patient up and giving 60% oxygen, maintaining the airway, and giving I.V. dexamethasone (20mg), I.V. frusemide (40mg) and possibly IV phenytoin. Emergency surgical bypass may be indicated. Prognosis is poor if a patient presents with advanced SVCO, and it may not be reversible with RT.

Management of SVCO is either with RT with steroid cover or with chemotherapy (for small-cell lung, lymphoma or testicular cancer.) RT is given with high dose steroids (e.g. dexamethasone 12mg per day) to prevent initial swelling and worsening of symptoms. Common regimes are 2000 cGy in 5 days, or 3000 cGy over 10 days. Improvement after RT or chemotherapy begins within 72 hours. Survival can be prolonged several months by treatment. Symptoms may recur, when high-dose steroids may produce a second remission, but it may become a terminal event requiring diamorphine to control dyspnoea and midazolam or other sedatives to control agitation.

SVC thrombosis is rare and usually suspected when SVCO does not respond to RT. It may occur as a complication of an infected IV catheter. It is diagnosed by CT scan or venogram and symptoms respond to anti-coagulation.

SWEATING

Heavy sweating occur in about 5% of cancer patients. Sweats occur most commonly in lymphomas, mesotheliomas and small cell cancer of the lung. Sweats are usually worse at night. They often occur in episodes, lasting days or weeks and then stopping for a time. Sweating is presumably due to tumour peptides acting on the hypothalamus (it has been observed that plasma exchange controls sweating in lymphoma). Exclude

- Infections
- Anxiety
- Thyrotoxicosis

Paracetamol is anti-pyretic and can help to reduce sweating in some patients.

NSAIDs such as indomethacin can reduce sweating, possibly because prostaglandins are involved in the physiology of the development of fever.

Propranolol 20-40mg 6 hourly can reduce sweating. It should not be given to patients with a history of asthma or heart failure.

Broad-spectrum antibiotics should be given if infection is suspected as a cause of sweating. Fever may not occur if the patient is on steroids.

General measures include regular washing, skin cooling with an electric fan and encouraging oral fluids to avoid dehydration.

TALKING WITH PATIENTS

What do patients want? Doctors are beginning to realize that patients want more than factual information; they are looking for emotional support and explanation and they often want to explore the questions Why me? Why now? Why this illness? In short patients want a doctor that listens. Patients want friendly professional interest that is sincere and sustained. The other essentials are honesty and encouragement.

Effective communication is a skill. Most complaints by patients about doctors concern communication problems. Clinical communication skills do not reliably improve from mere experience, but can be reliably taught and assessed. Highly structured programmes that identify, demonstrate, practise and evaluate skills are most effective. Video and audiotape review, role play and the use of standardized patients are effective teaching tools. Basic skills include listening (without premature closure) demonstrating empathy, open-ended questions, frequent summaries, clarification, negotiation and avoiding premature advice and reassurance. These skills need to be much more widely taught and assessed (*see Counselling*).

Telling the truth is essential, but truth, like medication, must be intelligently used, respecting its potential to help but also to harm. We must offer genuine opportunities to ask questions but must never give unrequested information, and bad news should be given skilfully (*see Explanation*). The longer-term benefits of knowing outweigh the short-term anguish of finding out. The fear of causing demoralization and despair often leads relatives (and sometimes professionals as well) to avoid the truth in the false hope that it will somehow protect the patient from distress. But unrealistic reassurance destroys trust and deprives the patient of opportunities to put their affairs in order, plan for their future care and their family's future, to deal with unfinished emotional business and to prepare for death. The opportunity to overcome fears and to retain some control often brings increased confidence.

Talking about prognosis can be either very helpful or very harmful, depending on how it is done. A discussion about prognosis must happen at the right time for the patient. The principles of breaking any bad news must be applied (*see Explanation*). Most patients reach a point where they would rather have more information than live with the uncertainty of not knowing (the hardest emotion to bear). Many fear that death will be sudden. It can reduce uncertainty and fear to explain "This illness will shorten your life, you have longer than days and weeks but I don't think you have years and years any more". Never guess about the precise length of time which causes fear as the date approaches and anyway will be inaccurate. Estimates of prognosis are usually inaccurate (and usually over-estimated) by hospice professionals. In a survey of 50 deaths the median estimate for survival was 8 weeks (range 1-28 weeks) but the median survival was in fact only 2 weeks (range 0-40weeks). (Palliative Medicine 1987; 1: 165-6).

Transactional analysis (TA) can provide a very useful framework for understanding professional-patient interactions. TA is based on the observation that all of us are 3 persons in one. We have 3 ego states, which can be called Parent, Adult and Child. TA looks at the content of each interaction. One part of me (Parent, Adult or Child) says something, and one part of you (Parent, Adult or Child) responds.

Most descriptions of communications with patients assume that every transaction is Adult-Adult, e.g. the patient requests information and the doctor or nurse responds by explaining something in a straightforward way. However the true situation is much more complex. First it is necessary to describe each of the ego states.

The Parent is the caring and nurturing part of us (derived from our own parental experiences). Ideally the Parent is affirming and sets clear boundaries of right and wrong, but can be over-protective and over-critical. The Parent in us says "I ought to" or "He ought to".

The Adult is the rational decision-maker in the here and now. The Adult in us says "These are the options".

The Child is creative and spontaneous but is also vulnerable and in need of support and can be selfish and manipulative. The Child in us says "I want to".

Many ill patients regress and need warmth, reassurance and touch and spend more time in their Child ego state ("What do you think I should do doctor"). This may prompt a Parent-type response from the carer ("What you must do is...."). This is a parallel transaction, (Child-Parent, Parent-Child) and in theory can go on for ever:

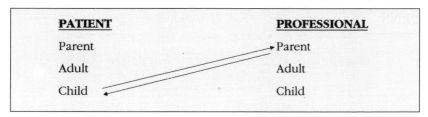

If a patient is being inappropriately dependent it may be necessary to challenge the pattern of the transaction, and reply in an Adult-Adult way (e.g. "What do you think might be best for you?"):

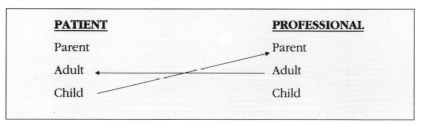

This is called a crossed transaction and stops communication, until the transaction is re-negotiated. The patient may then decide to continue this Adult-Adult transaction (e.g. "I think I need to start thinking about going home again for a while"). Or the patient may try to continue in a Child ego state ("I don't know, I'll have to ask my wife") or may switch and cross the transaction in a different way by suddenly using a Parent ego state to set up a challenge ("I thought you were supposed to be the doctor").

This model of interaction makes redundant the longstanding debate about whether a doctor should be simply a provider of information and expertize ("cold") or warm and supportive ("patronizing"). It is a question of balance, with different types of transaction being appropriate at different times. Transactions should be Adult-Adult most of the time, but there is an important place for other patterns of interaction.

A patient who is frightened and unable to make decisions may need to be allowed to regress to a Child state for a time, but at other times may need an Adult-Adult exchange of information.

Other patterns occur occasionally. Sometimes it is appropriate to lighten the atmosphere by sharing a joke (Child-Child transaction), since humour can be used to ventilate feelings and is about shared human experiences. Sometimes it can be helpful for a carer to demonstrate vulnerability by making a Child-comment ("I feel tired out today") allowing a patient the opportunity to be a Parent for a change, and narrowing the gap between the "healthy" carer and the "vulnerable" patient.

References:
Armstrong D. What do patients want? Br Med J 1991; 303: 261-2)
Simpson M et al. Doctor-patient communication: the Toronto consensus statement. Br Med J 1991; 303: 1385-7.
Gilhooly MLM et al. Truth telling with dying cancer patients. Palliative Medicine 1988; 2: 64-7.)

TENS

Transcutaneous electrical nerve stimulation (TENS) delivers electrical impulses to the skin from a small pulse generator, via skin electrodes. TENS was developed as a method of pain control after Melzack and Wall described the gate theory of pain control in 1967, which postulated that skin stimulation of large A fibres could reduce pain transmission to the spinal cord by C fibres.

Indications for TENS are mainly non-malignant pains:

- musculo-skeletal pains
- cervical spondylosis
- lumbar backache
- joint pains
- post-herpetic neuralgia

There are few studies of TENS for cancer pain. It may be helpful for some patients with bone pain, but is less useful for visceral or pelvic pain.

Mode of action: TENS stimulates the underlying sensory nerves and increases activity in the large A fibres, which reduces impulses in the smaller pain fibres (The Gate Theory of 1967) probably by releasing opioids in the dorsal horn.

Settings on the TENS machine:

- Amplitude 0-50 mAmperes
- Frequency 1-200 Hz (pulses per sec)
- Pulse duration 100-300 microseconds

Amplitude is the main control, and is increased until a distinct pulsation is felt. Avoid rapid increase, which can cause painful muscle contraction.

Frequency is often suggested in TENS instructions as 80 Hz to start with, but in fact is best set low, at 4 Hz, which means the amplitude of the stimulus has to be increased, to cause a distinct pulsation. Low frequency, high amplitude TENS produces a longer lasting effect.

Pulse duration is usually set at 200 microseconds, and only needs to be increased if large electrodes are used, which require a larger pulse duration to produce the same effect as small electrodes.

The wave form of the stimulus (square, spike, biphasic) is not important, as they all stimulate peripheral nerves to the same extent.

The electrodes are applied before the machine is switched on. A thin layer of gel is applied to cover the whole electrode surface. Insufficient gel may result in skin burns at higher amplitudes. The ideal electrode size is about 2 cm square, and they are placed close together but not touching. For larger areas 4 electrodes are needed (if the machine has 2 channels). Each channel is connected to 2 electrodes. Electrodes can be left on all day, and the machine switched on and off as required. Self-adhesive electrodes are easier to use as no jelly is needed.

The sites of electrode placement is best related to anatomically located acupuncture points. This is more effective than simply applying the electrodes to the painful areas. In theory, specific points can be chosen to stimulate spinal nerve roots, peripheral nerves, cutaneous nerves, muscles (motor points) and sympathetic nerves.

Duration of TENS should be no longer than 20 minutes twice a day, to avoid habituation. The nervous system tunes out a repetitive signal.

Multi-channel TENS has been developed to reduce the problem of habituation, which begins to occur after only 45 seconds of ordinary TENS, but does not seem to occur when several channels are stimulated randomly.

Further research is needed. Well designed studies are needed to establish the place of TENS in cancer patients, both for pain control and possibly to control other symptoms such as nausea, by using systemic acupuncture points.

Reference:
Librach SL Rapson LM, The Use of Transcutaneous Electrical Nerve Stimulation (TENS) for the Relief of Pain in Palliative Care, Palliative Medicine 1988; 2:15-20.

TERMINAL AGITATION

Terminal agitation is characterized by mental and physical agitation. It occurs in about 5% of dying people. The clinical picture can include:

- Restlessness
- Rambling speech
- Disorientation
- Loss of short-term memory
- Paranoid delusions
- Hallucinations
- Aggressive behaviour

A combined IM injection of the following drugs, given together, is usually effective within 30 minutes:

- Diamorphine Dose = 50% of 4 hourly oral morphine
- Hyoscine 0.4mg
- Chlorpromazine 50-200mg

Haloperidol (Serenace) 5-30mg, or methotrimeprazine (Nozinan) 50-200mg are alternatives to chlorpromazine. Resistance to medication is a feature of this condition, and some patients need high doses of sedatives. All these drugs (except chlorpromazine) can be used together in a subcutaneous infusion via a syringe pump (*see Subcutaneous infusions*).

Rectal diazepam (Stesolid enema) 10mg can provide useful additional sedation if the above is still not enough, or if rapid sedation is needed.

Indomethacin suppositories, 100mg 12 hourly, can be very helpful if the patient is still agitated on movement, due to painful bone metastases.

Sedation is indicated to relieve fear and distress and should always be given promptly if the patient is distressed by the agitation. It can always be reduced or stopped later, to assess whether the patient's mental state has calmed down. Exclude a full bladder and catheterize if necessary. Longterm sedation for several days before death is very occasionally unavoidable, in a psychotic or severely agitated patient, when reducing the medication results in a return of the distress.

The question of hydration (nasogastric or intravenous) then arises, since the patient may die of dehydration a few days before they would otherwise have died of their cancer. This may seem an academic point, but it can cause a great deal of concern for relatives and in a sedated patient the question of hydration should always be discussed with the family (*see Dehydration*).

TERMINAL PHASE

The Terminal phase can be defined as the period when day-to-day deterioration is occuring. There is weakness (sometimes profound), drowsiness, recumbency, poor appetite, organ failure and finally peripheral cyanosis. It is difficult to predict when the terminal phase will occur. Comfort is the priority at this stage and opioids and sedatives are used as necessary to achieve comfort. There is no evidence that drugs used to relieve distress hasten death, (but nor is death actively sought to achieve relief, which would be active euthanasia).

Causes of death in cancer are complex and often several factors are involved, including infection (pneumonia, septicaemia), organ failure (lung, heart, liver, kidney, brain), infarctions (lung, heart), haemorrhage (visceral, brain, external) and metabolic changes. The metabolic effects of tumours remain poorly understood. Several tumour-associated products have been described such as ectopic hormones, oncofetal antigens (CEA, AFP, beta-HCG), prostaglandins and angiogenesis factors, but their biological activity is far from understood.

Nursing care in the terminal phase may involve:

- Regular re-positioning or turning
- Mouth care

- Catheter or incontinence pads
- Eye drops

Specialized mattresses (*see Pressure sores*) can be useful to keep the patient comfortable. Mouth care can be done by the relatives, if they wish. Check for urinary retention which will cause restlessness, and insert an indwelling catheter if necessary (many of the drugs used have anti-cholinergic side-effects and may cause retention). Hypromellose eye-drops should be used if the eyelids are open in a semi-conscious patient, to prevent the eyes drying out or ulcerating. It is important to continue to talk to the patient and explain procedures both as a mark of respect and also because it is very supportive to relatives to see this happening.

Medication continues to be needed to control symptoms. 60% of patients can still swallow and take oral medication in the last 24 hours of life, but swallowing becomes tiring and difficult for some. Others prefer to avoid injections, when medication can often be given by spoon or syringe. Repeated injections can be avoided by means of a subcutaneous infusion (*see Subcutaneous infusions*).

Terminal agitation occurs in some patients as they die. Exclude a full bladder or rectum and consider strong sedation (*see Terminal agitation*).

Myoclonic jerking may be due to uraemia but can occur without, and may possibly be due on some occasions to high doses of morphine and phenothiazines. Rectal diazepam or SC midazolam are usually effective to control myoclonic twitching, but may not be adequate for severe myoclonus which may be controlled by a SC infusion of water soluble phenobarbitone 400-800mg per 24 hours (Dunlop RJ. Is terminal restlessness drug induced? Palliative Medicine 1989; 3: 65-66).

Bubbling (The "death rattle") is common and can be distressing to relatives, and is usually controlled with anti-cholinergics (*see Bubbling*).

Hydration is not indicated in the terminal phase. Hunger and thirst are not problems to the patient and artificial hydration or feeding are more likely to increase discomfort than to relieve it (*see Dehydration*).

Gastric atony can cause restlessness due to gastric distension. The patient has intermittent regurgitation of fluids and is semi-conscious. Nasogastric suction can be performed with little or no discomfort and the tube removed once the fluid is aspirated. This prevents large volumes being regurgitated at the time of death, which is distressing for relatives.

Warfarin should be stopped prior to the terminal phase if possible, or reversed with vitamin K. This prevents gastric bleeding and regurgitation of blood which is distressing for relatives (*see Bleeding*).

Family support around the time of death is very important. Feelings of confusion, grief, being out of place, anger, feeling left out, relief and guilt are all common. Ability to concentrate in this emotionally-charged situation is poor and relatives may need a suprising amount of guidance about straightforward decisions (e.g. how to get home) and about what it is appropriate to do (e.g. "Sit down by the bed, if you like, and hold his hand like this"). They may not think of making a rota for visiting, so that some can rest while others keep a vigil. They may need emotional support and guidance about practical needs (food, rest). Questions are often unasked (out of embarrassment at saying the wrong thing) and may include:

- Is he suffering?
- Can she hear?
- How long?
- Why does the breathing change?
- Why is the skin mottled?

All procedures (even simple ones) should be carefully explained.

The events around the time of death affect a family's future. One good memory can sometimes wipe away years of bad memories. Support at this stage is an effective form of preventive psychiatry (*see Family Support*).

Mode of death is usually with a period of unconsciousness, lasting hours to days, often with bronchopneumonia. Sudden deaths are usually due to a pulmonary embolus, (often as the patient is being moved) or massive haemorrhage, (usually internal, but occasionally external). Dying patients are not all comatose and about 10% remain orientated right up to the last few hours before death. Diagnosis of death involves confirming lack of pulse and respiration.

After the death relatives should be allowed to spend as long as they want with the dead person, and given the time and space to do what is important for them. Some may need time and guidance to decide what they do want to do. Relatives can be gently encouraged to view the body which facilitates the grieving process. Prayers at the bedside is strengthening for family and professionals.

Last offices are performed after a death. The body is washed as for a bed bath, as a mark of respect, and clean bedclothes put on. The body is straightened, the eyes closed and rings removed before rigor mortis occurs. Tubes and catheters are removed and wounds covered with adhesive plaster to prevent leakage. Pacemakers should be removed. If gastric contents are leaking the body may need to be tipped head-down for some time to allow drainage. The ankles are bandaged together. The face should normally be left uncovered and make-up is generally best avoided. The family may want to help with the last offices. Ask about special religious requirements, such as ritual washing, or the need to have certain rituals or ceremonies performed. It is best to discuss religious needs before the death occurs.

Post mortem examinations (autopsies) are an important way to improving our understanding of symptom control. Limited symptom-directed post-mortems may be acceptable to relatives and have clarified our understanding of some problems, for example, it has been found that severe dysphagia in patients with oropharyngeal cancers can occur with no demonstrable obstruction, due to extra-pharyngeal spread of malignancy and splinting of soft tissues, when dysphagia will respond to high dose steroids. Also some of the severe pains in head and neck cancers may be due to the peri-neural spread that has been recognized as typical of these tumours. Relatives may welcome a post mortem that will increase understanding of symptom control.

References:
Carter RL, The role of limited symptom-directed autopsies in terminal malignant disease. Palliative Medicine 1987; 1: 31-36.
Ashby M, Stofell B. Therapeutic ratio and defined phases: proposal of ethical framework for palliative care. Br Med J 1991; 302: 1322-24.
Lombard DJ, Oliver DJ, The use of opioid analgesics in the last 24 hours of life in patients with advanced cancer. Palliative Medicine 1989; 3: 27-29.
Ackworth A, Bruggen P. Family therapy when one member is on the death bed. Journal of Family Therapy 1985; 7: 379-385.

TESTICULAR CANCER

Testicular cancer causes 150 deaths per year in the UK. It only accounts for 1% of cancers in men, but is the commonest cancer in men aged 15-34. 50% are teratomas and 50% are seminomas. The cure rate is high, which makes it particularly difficult for the patients who progress to have advanced incurable disease.

Teratomas secrete high levels of a-feto-protein and chorionic gonadotrophin in 80% of cases. 10% have no palpable lump, when the primary can be visualized by testicular ultrasound scan. Metastases occur to para-aortic nodes and mediastinal nodes and to the lung (and to liver and CNS in far-advanced cases). Even with advanced disease 70% can now be cured by combined chemotherapy including cisplatin. Surgery may be needed to remove residual tumour masses.

Seminomas secrete only low levels of chorionic gonadotrophin. They are highly radio-sensitive, and most cases are cured with RT. Recurrent disease is unusual and 75% are still cured with chemotherapy.

Reference:
Br Med J 1992; 304: 1426-9.

THRUSH

Thrush (Candida) is a fungal infection. 70% of patients with advanced cancer develop oral thrush. Asymptomatic thrush is present in up to 50% of healthy adults. A survey of 140 terminally ill patients given weekly oral swabs (total swabs 510) showed thrush in 56% of all swabs, and in 89% of patients who had 6 or more swabs taken.

Steroids and antibiotics (especially together) predispose to thrush, and prophylaxis with nystatin should be considered.

Symptoms of oral thrush include:

- Sore lips
- Dry mouth
- Sore mouth
- Dysphagia (oesophageal)
- Hoarseness (laryngeal)

Soreness and dryness of the mouth occur commonly without thrush, as well as with it, and routine oral hygiene is important (*see Mouth Care*).

Signs of oral thrush are:

- Angular stomatitis
- Redness (atrophic variety)
- White plaques (pseudo-membraneous)

Inspect the tongue, lips, gums, throat, roof of the mouth and inside the cheeks. Some patients can have oral thrush with no symptoms. N.B. Staphylococcal infection can also produce white lesions in the mouth.

Oesophageal thrush can cause severe dysphagia, characterized by pain on swallowing hot drinks. It causes a typical tram-line pattern on barium swallow. Laryngeal thrush can cause hoarseness and is difficult to eradicate.

Anti-fungal agents include

- Polyenes (nystatin, amphotericin)
- Imidazoles (ketoconazole, clotrimazole, econazole)
- Triazoles (fluconazole, itraconazole)

Nystatin (Nystan) suspension, 1ml QID, is a contact agent, (it is not absorbed) and needs to be held in the mouth (with dentures out) and moved around the mouth with the tongue, before being swallowed. It is best used as a preventative measure, especially in patients on steroids or antibiotics. It is not effective for extensive thrush. In the survey mentioned above, no statistically significant improvement in symptoms or signs occured in the 43 patients with oral thrush treated with nystatin.

Ketoconazole (Nizoral), is the only well-absorbed imidazole. 200mg daily or BD as tablet or suspension, for 7 days. The symptoms usually begin to settle within 1-2 days. It can cause nausea and there is a slight risk (1 in 15000) of hepatitis.

Fluconazole (Diflucan) is a triazole. 50mg capsule a day is an alternative to ketoconazole, with fewer side-effects, and is widely used in AIDS. It is expensive.

Reference:
Finlay IG, Oral symptoms and Candida in the terminally ill, BMJ 1 March 1986; 292: 592-3.

UNKNOWN PRIMARY TUMOUR

Carcinomatosis due to an unknown primary tumour, means metastatic cancer, proven on histology, with no evidence of the primary tumour on routine investigations (including occult bloods in stools and prostatic acid phosphatase). It is seen in about 10% of hospice patients.

Presentation is usually with weight loss and weakness. Metastases may be found in lymph nodes, bone, liver or ascitic or pleural fluid (and occasionally skin or brain). It is obviously important that treatable tumours are not missed. Diagnosis should be based on histology as well as scans whenever possible.

Effective systemic treatment with chemotherapy or hormones may be possible if the primary carcinoma is from:

- Breast
- Prostate
- Lung (small cell)
- Ovary
- Thyroid

Therefore mammograms, CT scans, pelvic imaging in women, and thyroid scans should all be considered. Axillary nodes suggest an occult breast cancer, and tamoxifen should be considered. Malignant ascites may be from ovarian cancer which can respond for 1-2 years to chemotherapy. Multiple bone metastases in men may be treated with anti-androgen therapy in case it is an undetected prostatic cancer.

Anaplastic or poorly differentiated carcinomas should always prompt a careful review of the histology using specialized techniques (immunocytochemistry, electron microscopy, karyotyping and possibly hybridization for nucleic acids) because such tumours may in fact be lymphomas or germ cell tumours, which may be curable with chemotherapy. Plasma a-fetoprotein and HCG levels may be elevated in germ cell tumours.

Adenocarcinomas are usually from the lung or GI tract (stomach, pancreas, colon) at post mortem. Since there is no effective treatment for these tumours then invasive tests on the lung and bowel are not usually performed. A woman with metastatic adenocarcinoma should be given tamoxifen, in case it is due to an occult breast cancer.

Squamous cancer in cervical nodes suggests a primary is in the nasopharynx or thyroid (and thyroid tumours may be treatable with radio-iodine). A detailed ENT assessment is needed because surgery and RT can cure some ENT cancers. Squamous cancer in inguinal nodes suggests a primary in the perineum or perianal region.

Chemotherapy for carcinomatosis due to an unknown primary site is generally disappointing. Regimens based on doxorubicin or cisplatin are sometimes tried and 20-30% respond, but the effect is short-lived, toxicity is high and survival is not improved.

Prognosis is poor, with a median survival of only 5 months. The tumour spreads aggressively when the primary is still small and undetectable. At post-mortem most tumours are found to be in the lung or abdominal cavity (stomach, pancreas, liver or ovary).

Explanation often needs to be given more than once as to where the primary tumour might be, why further investigations are not being performed, and why no specific treatment is being given. Explanation can save a patient spending the last months of their life chasing further opinions.

Reference:
Bradley C, Selby P. In search of the unknown primary. Br Med J 1992; 304: 1065-6.

URINARY PROBLEMS

Urinary problems occur in about 20% of hospice patients. For difficult problems consider referral to either a consultant urologist or a specialist incontinence adviser.

Urinary infection is suggested by cloudiness of the urine together with one of the following: dysuria, frequency, incontinence, strong smell, pyrexia, loin or suprapubic pain, confusion. Urinary nitrites (detectable with a reagent strip) is a sensitive and specific bed-side test of urine infection, and a better indicator than protein, blood or symptoms. Culture urine and start an appropriate antibiotic. Continue antibiotics for several weeks if there is loin pain, suggesting pyelonephritis.

Urinary frequency is commonly due to:

- Infection
- Impacted faeces
- Excessive diuretics

Nocturnal frequency or incontinence can sometimes be improved by starting a diuretic in the morning, to alter the diurnal pattern of urine output. For male patients a urodom worn at night allows a good night's sleep. Nasal desmopressin 10-40 micrograms at bedtime will reduce urine production by the kidneys for 12 hours, and can occasionally be helpful. The dose must be adjusted to make sure the patient has a daytime urine output of at least 500ml (*see Diabetes insipidus*).

Urinary urgency (irritable bladder) can be due to local disease or damage to nerve pathways. Imipramine 10-50mg at night can be helpful. Propantheline, 15-30mg 8 hourly is an alternative anti-cholinergic. Oxybutinin (Ditropan) 5mg 2-4 times daily is a powerful anti-cholinergic and has calcium antagonist properties. It is useful if there is severe urgency or frequency due to an irritable bladder or bladder spasms.

Polyuria means large volumes of dilute urine, which causes thirst. The commonest cause is diabetes mellitus, less commonly it is due to hypercalcaemia and a rare cause is diabetes insipidus which is due to lack of anti-diuretic hormone from the pituitary gland and is treated with Desmopressin (*see Diabetes insipidus*).

Incontinence is best managed with an indwelling catheter, having excluded infection, impacted faeces or excessive diuretics. Alternatives to a catheter may be appropriate. A Self-adhesive urinary condom (Incontinence sheath, produced by Hollister Ltd) of the right size, worn at night, can help male patients disturbed by frequency or incontinence to get a good night's sleep. A penis pouch (Hollister) is used if the penis is retracted and a sheath cannot be fitted. The pouch adheres around the base of penis like a colostomy bag and drains into a tube and catheter bag. Disposable underpads may be sufficient for active patients with only slight incontinence. Continuous dribbling incontinence suggests a vesico-vaginal fistula. A urinary diversion procedure may be indicated, if the patient is fit enough for surgery (ileal conduit or uretero-sigmoidostomy). An alternative is the use of a vaginal prosthesis made of silicone, which incorporates a catheter (Green and Phillips 1986).

Stress incontinence, on coughing or straining, is usually due to a degree of prolapse, and can be controlled by inserting a vaginal ring pessary of the correct size. Atrophic vaginitis can cause urinary symptoms and can be treated with Dienoestrol cream, or with an oral oestrogen, such as oestradiol 1mg daily.

Bladder spasms cause severe suprapubic pain (*see Pain*).

Urinary retention or severe hesitancy usually require catheterization, to prevent painful urinary retention from occuring. It may be due to impacted faeces, anti-cholinergic drugs (tricyclics, chlorpromazine, hyoscine) or may be a late feature of spinal cord compression. Hesitancy may recur following treatment of either prostatic hypertrophy or prostatic cancer, and TURP (transurethral resection of the prostate) can then be repeated. A selective alpha-blocker can be used to relax urethral smooth muscle in prostatism and can improve urine flow. Indoramin (Baratol, Doralese) starting at 20mg BD, and increasing slowly by 20mg every 2 weeks to a maximum of 100mg daily in divided doses, can improve urine flow when there is prostatic obstruction, but care is needed, as hypotension can occur.

Discolouration of urine may be due to danthron (in co-danthramer and co-danthrusate) which causes red urine. Dark discolouration may be dehydration or bile staining (in jaundice) rather than blood.

Haematuria means blood in the urine. 1% Alum bladder irrigation, via a 3-way catheter, is the best treatment for heavy bladder haemorrhage in patients unfit for surgery (*see Bleeding*). Microscopic or light haematuria needs no action, other than excluding any infection. Reassure the patient and consider starting oral iron. Citrate bladder washouts can dissolve clots, and prevent clot retention. Bladder or renal haemorrhage may be controlled by radiotherapy if RT has not already been given in the past. Tranexamic acid (Cyclocapron) 500mg QID, can control mild haematuria, but the patient should be advised to increase fluid intake to prevent clot retention. Oral ethamsylate (Dicynene) 500mg QID enhances platelet adhesiveness and is excreted unchanged in urine, and may reduce light bleeding. Surgical options for bladder haemorrhage include total cystectomy, hydrostatic balloon distension (compressing the mucosa) or simply clot removal or cystoscopic laser. Renal embolization can be very effective for renal haemorrhage (*see Interventional radiology*).

Urethral catheterization is usually the best solution for incontinence or retention. A sialastic catheter should be used for long-term use, with a leg-bag for mobile patients. A leak around the catheter is an occasional problem, sometimes solved by changing to a smaller catheter (to increase urethral tone) or a smaller balloon. Debris or clots may be due to infection, but sometimes occur even after infection is treated, and bladder wash-outs using saline or citrate solution (which dissolves clots) can prevent blockage of the catheter. If a urethral stricture or vulval tumour prevents the passage of an ordinary catheter, a suprapubic catheter may be necessary.

The procedure of catheterization includes using a 14 FG (14mm circumference) Foley catheter initially, as smaller ones can curl up in the urethra at the prostatic narrowing. If there is difficulty passing it through the prostatic urethra use a larger size, 18-20 FG, which is firmer and more likely to part the lobes of the prostate. If the catheter fails to pass, or causes bleeding, then there is a stricture and a suprapubic catheter may be needed. If urine fails to flow initially the catheter tip may be blocked with the anaesthetic gel -- flush with sterile water. If inflating the balloon causes pain it is still in the urethra – deflate the balloon and insert the catheter further. Measure and record the amount of urine drained.

Female catheterization is usually straightforward, but if the urethra is difficult to locate it may be more posterior than normal and set in the anterior vaginal wall, when the left lateral position may be easier.

A 3-way catheter has an additional channel for irrigation, or a haematuria catheter can be used, which is strengthened to stop it collapsing when suction is applied to remove clots.

Intermittent catheterization can be useful alternative to an indwelling catheter in a relatively active patient who has difficulty emptying the bladder, e.g. due to a pelvic tumour that has damaged the lumbo-sacral plexus. A simple 10 FG Jacques catheter is used, and only men require lubricant. The catheter should be passed 4 times a day by the clock. Cleanliness is required, but not sterility. Rotate the catheter before removing and immerse in Milton's between use.

A suprapubic catheter is only rarely needed for retention if a urethral catheter cannot be passed because of a urethral stricture or vulval tumour. The bladder must be distended with urine and there must be no haematuria. There are several types of catheter. The Bonnano (Becton Dickinson) is easy to insert, being of narrow gauge at 6 FG having an inner insertion trocar. It is inserted in the midline, 3 cm above the pubic symphysis. Infiltrate with local anaesthetic first down to the bladder, until urine is drawn back, then use a pointed scalpel to make a stab wound. Follow the manufacturer's instructions. The distal end has a preformed pigtail memory curve, to prevent it going down the urethra. The flange is sutured to the skin.

If the bladder is not distended enough at the time of insertion, there is a risk of puncturing a loop of bowel, but with a fine 6FG catheter there is little risk of peritonitis – start metronidazole and a cephalosporin, and observe the patient for 24 hours. If the urine is blood-stained then if a suprapubic catheter is needed a wide-bore 22 FG catheter has to be inserted by open cystotomy.

VULVAL CANCER

Vulval cancers cause around 500 deaths per year in the UK. They are squamous and present with pruritus, pain, ulceration or discharge. There is usually a history of dystrophic skin changes. Diagnosis is by biopsy.

Radical excision is the treatment of choice. Skin grafting is not usually needed, due to the laxity of the skin. If inguinal nodes are involved 5 year survival falls to 40% (20% with pelvic nodes). If surgery is not possible palliative radiotherapy can reduce pain and ulceration, but vulval skin tolerates the acute RT skin reaction poorly.

Problems in advanced cancer of the vulva include:

- Ulceration
- Malignant nodes (pain, bleeding)
- Lymphoedema
- Hypercalcaemia

WEAKNESS

Weakness means loss of muscle power or lack of energy. It is the commonest symptom in patients with advanced cancer and is a problem for at least 80% of patients. However, a <u>careful history</u> is needed, because by "weakness" the patient may in fact mean immobility due to pain, lethargy (depression) or dyspnoea.

Generalized weakness is usually due to progression of malignant disease, but reversible causes should be remembered:

- Poor sleep
- Infection
- Anaemia
- Drugs (hypotensives, baclofen)
- Hypercalcaemia
- Hypokalaemia (diuretics, steroids)
- Parkinson's disease,
- Diabetes
- Hypothyroidism

<u>Hypotensive drugs</u> can often be stopped, because blood pressure falls in advanced illness as weight falls.

Sudden worsening of weakness suggests infection (thrush, urinary, chest), arrythmia, adrenal failure or hypokalaemia. <u>Arrythmias</u> can be caused by invasion of the right atrium by tumour. ECG is needed. Atrial tachycardias are usually controlled by verapamil and digoxin. <u>Adrenal failure</u> due to adrenal metastases (can be confirmed by a Synacthen test – ACTH does not increase plasma cortisol levels. It responds to steroids. <u>Hypokalaemia</u> can be due to ectopic ACTH (small cell lung cancer) treated with metyrapone, 250mg-1g 6 hourly, (which blocks the adrenals) plus replacement steroids.

Localized weakness may be due to:

- Brain metastases
- CVA (sudden onset)
- Cord compression (both legs)
- Malignant nerve damage (painful)
- Peripheral neuropathy (foot drop)
- Nerve palsy (wrist drop)

Nerve palsies in the arm are relatively common, especially if a weak patients spend a lot of time in a chair with hard arm-rests. Radial nerve palsy is due to pressure on the inside of the upper arm, e.g. sleeping with the arm in an awkward position. It causes wrist drop with little sensory loss, and the patient needs a wrist splint for 3-6 weeks until it recovers. Ulnar nerve palsy is usually due to pressure at the elbow from unpadded arm-rests, as the ulnar nerve passes close to the skin surface on the medial side of the elbow. It causes tingling and weakness in the 4th and 5th fingers.

Proximal leg weakness causes difficulty climbing stairs and standing up from a chair. It is usually due to a steroid myopathy but can also be caused by polymyositis or the Lambert-Eaton myasthenic syndrome (see below).

Peripheral neuropathy occurs in about 2% of patients with advanced cancer and is a non-metastatic manifestation of malignancy. It causes progressive glove and stocking sensory loss, loss of vibration sense and ankle reflexes and weakness of dorsiflexion of the foot. There is usually a mixed sensory and motor loss. Pure sensory loss is associated with small cell lung cancer. Nerve conduction studies confirm the type of neuropathy. There may be a painful burning dysaesthetic pain which may respond to amitriptyline or valproate. (Reference: Grant R. Non-metastatic manifestations of malignancy: neurological. Palliative Medicine 1989; 3: 181-188).

The Lambert-Eaton myasthenic syndrome occurs in around 3% of patients with small cell lung cancer. It causes proximal leg weakness and absent reflexes which re-appear after a sustained muscular contraction. Dryness of the mouth can occur due to autonomic neuropathy. It is commoner than paraneoplastic neuropathy and myopathy. It is due to tumour antibodies that cross-react with antigens at the motor nerve endings. (Similar cross-reactions may explain other paraneoplastic phenomena such as neuropathy and visual failure.) It may improve partially with steroids but responds specifically to 3,4-diaminopyride (DAP) which enhances neuromuscular transmission, at a starting dose 10mg TID, increasing to 30mg TID. DAP is available on a named patient basis from the Radcliffe Infirmary, Oxford. OX2 6HE (Reference: Palliative Medicine 1992; 6: 9-17).

Management of weakness focuses on helping the patient adjust physically and psychologically, and involves:

- Physiotherapy
- Occupational therapy (OT)
- Counselling

Physiotherapy is very beneficial in over 50% of hospice patients. Exercise seems the natural antidote to weakness, and it is often possible to restore or improve mobility, and to maintain independence. This frequently raises morale.

Occupational Therapy can be invaluable in helping the patient adjust to weakness, make adaptions to their home and lifestyle, and in overcoming the problem of boredom.

Counselling is essential. Psychological adjustment is usually more difficult than physical adjustment, and involves a process of grieving for the independence that has been lost. This needs time and talking. Explanation can help. Strength is limited, therefore periods of activity need to be alternated with periods of rest. Periods of rest often need to be "prescribed". Encourage the patient to develop realistic short-term goals (*see Counselling*).

A comment by a patient with Motor Neurone Disease is also relevant to many patients with advanced cancer: "An understanding of my unusual tiredness is very important. This illness needs rest during the day and lots of sleep at night. Over a period of time I have come to recognize within myself waves of energy, which are followed by long periods of exhaustion. Things can be tackled while my energy lasts which should not be attempted once the exhaustion has set in".

Drugs cannot restore strength. Dexamethasone 4mg daily can improve appetite and give a feeling of well-being in some patients. Blood Transfusion does not restore strength, and is only indicated for specific symptoms of anaemia (*see Anaemia*).

Visitors can be a dilemma for some weak patients. The support is welcome, but too many visitors can be very exhausting. It can be helpful for the patient or family to be able to say "The doctor says visiting must be limited" (e.g. only one visitor per morning or afternoon, and only to stay 10 minutes). A rota for visiting can be helpful. A rota allows visiting to be spaced out, so the patient is supported without being exhausted. It can also prevent the family getting exhausted. The ideal visitor is punctual, smiles, listens well, offers realistic encouragement, doesn't talk too much, communicates with the nurses, offers and delivers practical help and rarely stays longer than 10 minutes!

Further Reading:
Lichter I. Review article: Weakness in terminal illness. Palliative Medicine 1990; 4: 73-80.

WEIGHT LOSS

Weight loss occurs in almost all patients with advanced cancer. Prognosis is shortened by weight loss at any stage of the illness. Cachexia (profound weight loss) occurs in 20%. It happens despite reasonable food intake. It can occur with any tumour (most commonly lung, gut and ovary).

Tumour metabolism is extremely inefficient – a tumour weighing less than 2% body weight can utilize 40% of a patient's calorie intake. This has led to the concept of some tumours acting as a "nitrogen trap" – enabling the tumour to enlarge as the rest of the body is wasting. Some malignant tumours secrete peptides (such as "cachectin") which increase basal metabolic rate.

Management of weight loss involves:

- Explanation
- Dietary advice
- Physiotherapy
- Counselling

Explanation may be needed. Relatives may feel intensive feeding will help. But weight loss is due to cancer, not usually poor diet and intensive feeding does not improve weight or prolong survival. Sedentary individuals only need 1500 calories per day.

Dietary advice can be important psychologically. Consider referral to a dietician (*see Anorexia and Diet*).

Physiotherapy can help improve mobility (walking or transfering). Relatives may need teaching techniques of lifting and turning to protect skin over bony prominences.

Counselling can help. Weight loss can be frightening. "I'm wasting away, soon there will be nothing left". The real issue may be dying rather than weight loss. An altered body shape can be psychologically distressing, because the person may no longer recognize themselves. Photographs can help in adjusting to a new body image. Old photographs show carers how the patient still thinks of themselves. New family photographs can demonstrate that a person is still part of the family circle.

New clothes, that fit, can be a great boost to morale. Other problems include loose dentures and loose spectacles. Dentures can be relined by a dentist and loose spectacles can easily be adjusted to fit. Avoid routine weighing. Weight loss is inevitable. Weighing serves no useful purpose and can be demoralizing (*see Counselling*).

APPENDIX 1 - USEFUL EQUIPMENT

The correct equipment can greatly improve patient care and can ease the burden for carers. The following is a checklist of commonly used equipment, followed by individual items of equipment that we have found to be especially useful at Cynthia Spencer House. I am grateful to Sister Jo Warcaba for her help with this section.

Mobility aids include:

- Appropriate footwear
- Appropriate splinting
- Home adaptions (handrails, ramps, stairlift)
- Walking stick or tripod
- Walking frame
- Rollator (walking frame with wheels)
- Raised toilet seat
- Wheelchair (*see Rehabilitation*)

Living aids for day-to-day comfort include:

- High-backed chair
- Recliner chair
- Chair lift
- Chair cushions
- Non-slip mats
- Bath seat
- Commode

Eating or drinking equipment for weak patients:

- Shaped cutlery (combined spoon and knife)
- Non-slip jelly mats
- Plate guards
- 2-handled beakers
- Flexible straws
- Flask (hot\cold drinks)

Kitchen equipment that is useful in preparing food:

- High kitchen stool (to lean on)
- High trolley (to move things)
- Liquidizer
- Microwave
- Ice maker

Skin care and pressure reducing aids include:

- Chair cushion (e.g. Roho)
- Heel and elbow pads (e.g. Spenco)
- Special mattress cover (e.g. foam Pro-pad)

- Specialized mattress (e.g. Pegasus)
- Jelly cushions for bath and hoist

Bed comfort can be increased by the use of:

- Light bedding (e.g. Duvet)
- Trapeze
- Leg cradle
- V-pillow
- Spenco mattress
- Heel\elbow pads
- Tissues and basin
- Back rest eg Matchett bag (see below)

Incontinence aids:

- Bedpans
- Urine bottles
- Incontinence sheathes
- Penis pouches
- Catheter bags
- Plastic drawsheets
- Commode

Nursing equipment that is useful includes:

- 15 ml free-standing medicine spoon
- Foam mouth swabs
- Handling slings
- Hoist
- Bath seat

Symptom control equipment

- Drug card (*see Prescribing*)
- Portable syringe pump
- Nebulizer
- TENS machine
- Compression sleeve for lymphoedema.
- Drug dispenser

Quality of life for a bedbound patient can be enhanced by:

- Bed table and bedside light
- Electric fan
- Call bell\hand bell
- Flexible call bell for weak patients
- Remote-control TV and video
- Portable telephone

Useful individual items of equipment are described below, with addresses of manufacturers. If you know of any others I would be pleased to know to add to the list for a future edition.

Syringe pumps and infusion sets for subcutaneous infusions:
Graseby Medical Ltd
Colonial Way
Watford, Herts
England WD2 4LG
Tel: 0923 246434

Foam mouthswabs that are more effective than cotton swabs and helpful for mouthcare for patients unable to use a toothbrush:
Anglia Vale Medical
Unit 6
Lancaster Way business complex
Ely, Cambridgeshire
England CB6 3NW
Tel: 0353 666195

Bocasan mouthwash is useful for removing debris or coating from the tongue and mouth, but the patient must be able to co-operate as it must be held in the mouth for 2 minutes and not swallowed.
Oral-B laboratories Ltd
Gatehouse Road
Aylesbury
Buckinghamshire
England HP19 3ED

15ml free-standing plastic spoon is much easier to use than the plastic cup for some patients on liquid medication.
Medipost UK Ltd
17 Surrey Close
Granby Industrial Estate
Weymouth
Dorset
England DT14 9TY
Tel: 0305 760750

Incontinence sheaths and penis pouches for male patients avoid the need to insert a catheter. The incontinence sheaths are in 4 sizes. The pouches are used for patients with a retracted penis and fit like a colostomy bag over the penis.
Hollister Ltd
43 Castle St
Reading
England RG1 7SN
Tel: 0734 775545

Patient handling slings slide under a patient more easily than hands and arms, and reduce friction and shearing forces that contribute to pressure sores.

> MEDesign Ltd
> Freepost
> Southport
> England
> PR8 1BR
> Tel: 0704 542373

Pro-pad foam mattress, chair cushions and plastic covers are very comfortable for patients. They are relatively inexpensive and the compartments of foam disperse skin pressure and allow skin ventilation.

> Medical Support Systems
> 23 Argyle Way
> Cardiff
> England CF5 5NJ
> Tel: 0222 595425

Jelly cushions for the bath or hoist chair are very comfortable for the frail patient being moved and bathed.

> SUMED
> Beaumont Close
> Banbury
> Oxfordshire
> Tel: 0295 270499

Roho Air Flotation Cushions are very effective in preventing pressure sores, especially for patients who spend a long time in a wheelchair. They are inflated with a pump. They are more expensive than foam cushions and are difficult to clean. Suppliers in the UK are:

> Raymar
> PO Box 16
> Fairview Estate
> Reading Road
> Henley-on-Thames RG9 1LL
> Tel: 0491 578446

Machett bags are shaped bean bags that are very useful for positioning weak patients. They come in a variety of shapes, and are useful as back rests in bed, arm rests for lymphoedematous arms, cushions for foot stools etc. They are available from:

> Cuneiform
> The Old Post Office
> Weasenham Rd
> Great Massingham
> Norfolk PE32 2EY

Pegasus bi-wave or airwave mattresses are very useful for more immobile patients to help prevent pressure sores. The bi-wave is placed over a mattress, the airwave replaces the existing mattress and is more effective but more expensive. Alternating inflation and deflation of air cells periodically reduces skin pressure.

> Pegasus House
> Kingscroft Court, Havant
> Hampshire, England PO9 1LS
> Tel: 0705 451444

Compression pumps can be helpful in some cases of lymphoedema and are available from Talley or Centromed. Suppliers of Talley are:

> Chattanooga UK Ltd.
> Goods Rd
> Belper
> Derbyshire DE5 1UU
> Tel: 077382 6993\4

The address of Centromed Ltd is:

> Unit 5, Stafford Close
> Fairwood Industrial Park
> Ashford
> Kent TN23 2TT
> Tel: 0233 628018

A hand-held communicator very useful for communicating with some deaf patients, and is a portable amplifier for the voice with an attached ear-piece for the patient. The Contacta model HH\1 is very effective, available from:

> TVM (Manchester LTD)
> 9 Bloom St
> Salford
> Lancashire
> Tel: 061-834-2659

Lightwriter communication aids are very useful for patients with Motor Neurone Disease who have lost their speech but can still operate a keyboard. Suppliers:

> Toby Churchill Ltd.
> 20 Panton ST
> Cambridge. CB2 1HP
> Tel: 0223 316117

Environmental control systems (POSSUM) are useful to some patients with advanced Motor Neurone Disease. They are computerized systems that control a patient's environment from a single switch.

> Possum Controls Ltd
> Middlegreen Rd
> Langley
> Slough
> Berkshire SL3 6DF
> Tel: 0753 579234

APPENDIX 2 – USEFUL DRUGS

The following 41 drugs are used in hospice medicine and are very useful in routine symptom control. They are listed here for information and discussed in detail elsewhere.

Paracetamol, 1g 4 hourly, is useful for mild pains and tension headache.

Co-proxamol (Distalgesic) 2 tablets 4 hourly, is useful for moderate pains which are not severe enough to warrant morphine.

Morphine solution (Oramorph) is the best strong analgesic available for continuous cancer pain, (visceral or soft tissue pain). It is prescribed 4 hourly. Oramorph solution is available in 2 strengths 10mg in 5ml, and 20mg in 1ml. Sevredol tablets are an alternative for 4 hourly morphine (10mg and 20mg both scored and easily halved).

Slow-release morphine (MST, SRM-Rhotard) is useful after a patient has been stabilized on 4 hourly morphine. (10mg yellow, 15mg green, 30mg purple, 60mg orange, 100mg grey, 200mg blue). 90% pf patients need a dose in the range 10–200mg BD, but occasionally a patient may require very high doeses in the range of 2000–3000mg BD.

Diamorphine injections are useful because it is very soluble (400mg dissolves in 1ml). The equi-analgesic dose of diamorphine injection is half the oral morphine dose.

Lactulose (Duphalac) 20-30mg TID is a bowel softener that should be combined with senna tablets 1-2 BD, to prevent constipation in patients on analgesics.

Co-danthramer forte suspension is a useful strong oral laxative.

Fybogel 1 sachet daily or BD is a bulking agent useful for patients with a rectal discharge or for regulating colostomy function.

Naproxen (Naprosyn) 250-500mg 12 hourly is useful for bone pain due to metastases, available as tablets, solution or suppositories.

Indomethacin (Indocid) is the strongest NSAID available and useful for severe bone pain not responding to other NSAIDs.

Dexamethasone (Decadron) is used as the strong steroid of choice for anorexia or symptoms due to compression.

Ranitidine (Zantac) is used to treat dyspepsia or protect the stomach in patients on NSAIDs.

Nystatin (Nystan) 1ml 4 hourly is routinely used to prevent thrush.

Ketoconazole (Nizoral) 200mg daily or BD is used to treat severe symptomatic thrush.

Frusemide (Lasix) 40mg daily is used to treat troublesome ankle swelling due to fluid retention.

Spironolactone (Aldactone) 100-200mg BD is used to prevent the recurrence of ascites.

Metolozone (Metenix-5) 5-10mg daily is a powerful diuretic, when added to frusemide, for refractory oedema.

Metoclopramide (Maxolon) 10-20mg TID is a useful anti-emetic that causes no drowsiness. It is also useful to control hiccups. It can be given subcutaneously.

Cyclizine (Valoid) 50mg 8 hourly is a useful first-line anti-emetic. It can be given subcutaneously.

Haloperidol (Serenace) 1.5mg prevents nausea in patients started on morphine. Higher doses, 3-5mg BD, is useful in treating anxiety or agitation.

Chlorpromazine (Largactil) 25-50mg 8 hourly is useful for agitated patients who also require some sedation, and is useful for severe insomnia, given with a hypnotic. It cannot be given subcutaneously due to skin irritation.

Methotrimeprazine (Nozinan) is a powerful phenothiazine that can be given subcutaneously, 75-150mg per 24 hours, and is a powerful anti-emetic or useful in terminal agitation.

Temazepam 10-60mg at night is a short acting sleeping pill that is suitable for most patients.

Amitriptyline (Tryptizol) 25-150mg at night, is an anti-depressant that is also used to control nerve pain that has a burning element.

Dothiepin (Prothiaden) 50-150mg at night is a sedative anti-depressant with fewer anti-cholinergic side-effects than amitripyline.

Lofepramine (Gamanil) 70mg BD is a less sedating anti-depressant and has fewer anti-cholinergic side-effects than amitriptyline.

Lorazepam (Ativan) 0.5-1mg BD is a useful anxiolytic that is shorter acting than diazepam.

Midazolam (Hypnovel) is used in a subcutaneous infusions to control twitching (multifocal myoclonus), seizures, muscle stiffness, anxiety and terminal agitation. Dose range over 24 hours is 10-120mg. It can be mixed in an infusion with diamorphine, haloperidol, cyclizine, methotrimeprazine or hyoscine.

Diazepam enema (Stesolid) 10mg PR is useful in the emergency control of seizures or terminal agitation.

Hyoscine hydrobromide 0.4mg 4 hourly IM or SC is used to control terminal bubbling.

Hyoscine butylbromide (Buscopan) 40-80mg per 24 hours subcutaneously is used to control colic in intestinal obstruction.

Metronidazole (Flagyl) tablets and gel are used to control smell from anaerobic infections.

Terfenadine (Triludan) 60mg BD is a useful antihistamine for itching that causes little drowsiness.

Colestipol (Colestid) 5g sachet 1-2 times a day reduces itching in patients with partial biliary obstruction.

Tranexamic acid (Cyclokapron) 500mg QID is useful to control bleeding.

Topical adrenaline 1 in 1000 is useful to control superficial capilliary bleeding.

Oxybutinin (Ditropan) 5mg BD to QID is useful to control bladder spasms.

Pamidronate (Aredia) 30-90mg IV is used to control hypercalcaemia.

Ondansetron (Zofran) 8mg TID is a 5HT3 antagonist and is a powerful anti-emetic mainly used to prevent chemotherapy-induced vomiting.

Octreotide (Sandostatin) 300 micrograms per 24 hours by SC infusion can be used to treat severe diarrhoea or intractable vomiting. It is an analogue of somatostatin, which is a hypothalamic peptide.

Desmopressin (DDAVP) inhibits urine production by the kidneys and is useful in nocturnal frequency as well as diabetes insipidus. A starting dose of 100–200 micrograms orally at night is safe, the effect lasting about 12 hours.

INDEX